The Mindful Path Navigating Mental Health Challenges with Resilience and Compassion

Emily Reynolds

Copyright © [2023]

Title: The Mindful Path Navigating Mental Health Challenges with Resilience and Compassion

Author's: Emily Reynolds

All rights reserved. No part of this publication may be reproduced, stored in a retrieval system, or transmitted in any form or by any means, electronic, mechanical, photocopying, recording, or otherwise, without the prior written permission of the publisher or author, except in the case of brief quotations embodied in critical reviews and certain other non-commercial uses permitted by copyright law.

This book was printed and published by

ISBN:

For permission to reproduce any of the material in this book.

Table of content

Chapter name   **Page No**

1. A Primer on Mindfulness and Mental Health — 1
2. Challenges in Mental Health: A Better Understanding — 17
3. What You Need to Know About Mindfulness — 32
4. Strengthening Resistance — 45
5. Practising Kindness to Oneself — 65
6. Mindful Interaction and Communication — 85
7. Mindfulness-Based Stress Reduction — 105
8. Using Meditation to Recover from Trauma — 125
9. The Effects of Mindfulness on Individuals' Psychological Health — 146
10. Beyond the Textbook: Maintaining Your Meditation Practise — 169

Chapter 1:
A Primer on Mindfulness and Mental Health

1.1- Defining mental health

The state of one's mental health is intricate and multifaceted. It is vital to our survival and affects all aspects of our being: emotionally, mentally, and socially. Understanding the many facets of mental health and the importance of doing so will be the focus of this chapter.

Mental Health: A Spectrum

Like physical health, mental health can be on a range. One end of the mental health spectrum represents people who are emotionally stable, have high levels of resilience, and know why they're here on Earth. Mental health diseases, on the other hand, might vary in severity. Most people are in the middle, and they will likely experience some degree of mental ups and downs over the course of their life.

Realise that mental wellness is not an either/or proposition. You can be in diverse states of mental health just as you are in varying states of physical health. Mental health issues are an inevitable aspect of being human, and this spectrum helps us see that.

The Value of Emotional Well-Being

We should care about our mental health because.... The answer can be found in how significantly it affects our standard of living as a whole. Some of the many reasons why mental health is crucial include:

1 Emotional and Physical Health

The state of our emotions is an indicator of our psychological well-being. Emotions like joy, sorrow, anger, and fear arise as a result of our interactions with the world. When our mental health is good, we are able to recognise and deal with these feelings. Our ability to deal with life's difficulties is hindered by our emotional responses, which can become either overpowering or repressed when our mental health is in decline.

2 - Mental Processes

Memory, focus, problem-solving, and decision-making are just few of the cognitive talents that are affected by our mental health. When our mental health is strong, we are better able to take in new information, process it, and use that knowledge to guide our decision-making. On the flip side, mental health concerns might hinder these capabilities, making it harder to carry out routine duties.

Relationships, No. 3:

Strong bonds require two people to listen attentively, empathise, and trust one another. How we connect with others is heavily influenced by our mental health. Being emotionally stable and resilient strengthens our capacity to connect with others. However, untreated mental health concerns can put a strain on interpersonal connections and make it harder to make new ones.

Physical Fitness 4

Both mental and physical health are intertwined and interdependent. For instance, studies have connected long-term stress with heart disease, immune system dysfunction, and gastrointestinal difficulties. Taking care of your mental health is crucial to your overall health and happiness.

5. Effectiveness and Satisfaction

Productivity and a sense of meaning in life are both affected by our mental health. When our minds are strong, we are more able to fully participate in life. To add to our sense of accomplishment, we are now better able to direct our efforts towards worthwhile aims.

The Stigma of Mental Illness

There is still a substantial stigma attached to issues of mental health, despite the significance of addressing them. Discrimination, prejudice, and reluctance to seek treatment are all possible outcomes of stigma. Many people with mental health problems may therefore avoid discussing their problems or put off getting help.

Misconceptions, fear, and societal attitudes contribute to the stigma that exists in the field of mental health. It can make people feel even more ashamed and alone, which makes it harder for them to seek help. The first step towards improving everyone's mental health is eliminating the associated stigma and encouraging open dialogue on the topic.

The Effects of Social and Cultural Factors

Culture and society play a role in determining an individual's mental health. The ways in which people understand and talk about their mental health can be influenced by cultural ideas and expectations. There may be a greater emphasis on the well-being of the group in some cultures and on the well-being of the individual in others. Effectively addressing mental health issues requires an appreciation of the cultural and socioeconomic environment in which they occur.

The Complicated Nature of Mental Illness

There is a wide spectrum of mental health illnesses, each with its own set of symptoms and obstacles. Disorders of the mind that are very prevalent include:

Anxiety Disorders, Number One

Excessive worry and terror characterise anxiety disorders such generalised anxiety disorder, social anxiety disorder, and panic disorder. Physical symptoms, such as heart palpitations and shortness of breath, can arise from these disorders and make daily life difficult.

2 Emotional Disturbances

Conditions like sadness and manic-depressive mania are categorised as mood disorders. Both depression and bipolar illness are conditions that alter a person's emotional state, often causing bouts of severe sadness or elation.

Third, PTSD (Post-Traumatic Stress Disorder).

Combat, accidents, or sexual assault are just some of the traumatic situations that can trigger PTSD. Flashbacks, nightmares, and heightened vigilance are all possible side effects.

Eating Disorders, Number Four

Anorexia nervosa, bulimia nervosa, and other eating disorders are characterised by destructive patterns of thinking and behaving around food, self-perception, and weight. The effects on one's body and mind can be devastating.

Disorders Related to Substance Abuse

Substance use disorders stem from excessive drinking or drug use that eventually leads to dependency and distress.

Number Six: Schizophrenia

Schizophrenia is a severe mental illness that causes sufferers to experience disorganised thought processes, hallucinations, and a breakdown in their ability to interact socially.

Personality Disorders, 7

Persistent patterns of behaviour, thought, and interpersonal connections that differ from cultural standards are characteristic of personality disorders such borderline and narcissistic personality disorders.

Those who suffer from mental illness should not be judged on their own moral fibre. They represent medical disorders that, with the correct help and care, can be treated and controlled.

Finding Resources and Assistance

You or a loved one must get professional aid and emotional backing if you are experiencing mental health problems. Therapists, counsellors, and psychiatrists are just few of the experts in the field of mental health who have the education and experience to properly evaluate, diagnose, and treat their patients. They are able to assist people in regaining their mental health by providing them with direction, treatment, and medication if necessary.

Numerous self-help tactics and tools exist to promote mental health in addition to professional assistance. Among these are:

Practises of self-care include things like exercise, meditation, and hobbies that help one unwind and feel better emotionally.

- Social networks: asking for and receiving comfort and understanding from those you know and care about.
Accessing credible online websites, books, and articles that present knowledge and coping strategies for mental health difficulties is a key component of online resources.
When in need of emergency assistance, calling a crisis hotline or a support group is a good option.

Concluding Remarks

When we are emotionally, cognitively, relationally, and physically well, we are said to be whole. It's relative, and everyone has ups and downs in their mental health at different times.

Despite its importance, the stigma associated with mental health might prevent some people from getting the treatment they need. It is crucial to understand the cultural and societal background of mental health in order to properly address these issues.

Mental health issues are very variable and multifaceted problems. One of the most important things you can do for your mental health is to reach out for assistance of some kind.

Mindfulness is a potent technique that we will examine in the next chapters.

 coping with mental health issues, strengthening one's mental fortitude, and expanding one's capacity for empathy. Mindfulness is the first step on a lifelong path to improved emotional health and happiness.

1.2- The importance of mindfulness in mental well-being

The Importance of Mindfulness in Mental Well-Being

Mental well-being is a fundamental aspect of our overall health and quality of life. It encompasses our emotional, psychological, and social well-being and plays a pivotal role in how we perceive and interact with the world around us. To nurture and enhance our mental well-being, it's essential to explore the profound significance of mindfulness—a practice that has gained increasing recognition for its transformative effects on mental health.

Understanding Mindfulness

Before delving into the importance of mindfulness in mental well-being, let's clarify what mindfulness entails. At its core, mindfulness is a state of focused awareness on the present moment. It involves paying deliberate and non-judgmental attention to our thoughts, emotions, bodily sensations, and the surrounding environment. Mindfulness encourages us to observe our inner experiences with acceptance and without the need to change them.

Mindfulness has its roots in ancient Eastern practices, particularly in Buddhism, where it was cultivated as a means to attain inner peace and enlightenment. Over the past few decades, mindfulness has gained widespread recognition in Western psychology and medicine as a powerful tool for promoting mental well-being.

The Mind-Body Connection

One of the key reasons why mindfulness is crucial for mental well-being lies in the intricate connection between the mind and the body. The mind and body are not separate entities; they constantly interact and influence each other. Therefore, when we nurture our mental well-being through mindfulness, we are also benefiting our physical health and vice versa.

Mindfulness practices, such as meditation and deep breathing, can activate the body's relaxation response. This response counters the effects of the "fight or flight" stress response, which, when chronically activated, can lead to a range of physical and mental health issues, including anxiety, depression, and cardiovascular problems.

By reducing stress and promoting relaxation, mindfulness can help lower blood pressure, improve sleep quality, boost the immune system, and alleviate chronic pain. These physical benefits contribute to an overall sense of well-being and vitality.

Emotional Regulation

Emotions are a central component of our mental well-being. Mindfulness equips us with valuable tools for understanding, managing, and even transforming our emotions. When we practice mindfulness, we become more attuned to our emotional responses and gain the ability to observe them without immediate judgment or reaction.

This non-judgmental awareness of our emotions can prevent us from becoming overwhelmed by them. Rather than being carried away by waves of anger, anxiety, or sadness, we learn to ride them like a surfer on the ocean. This increased emotional regulation can lead to reduced reactivity and impulsivity, allowing us to respond to life's challenges with greater clarity and composure.

Furthermore, mindfulness can foster positive emotions and a greater sense of well-being. By cultivating gratitude, compassion, and joy through mindfulness practices, we can shift our emotional balance towards positivity, even in the face of adversity.

Cognitive Benefits

Our cognitive abilities are deeply intertwined with our mental well-being. Mindfulness has been shown to enhance various cognitive functions, including attention, memory, and problem-solving skills. When we practice mindfulness, we exercise and strengthen the prefrontal cortex—the part of the brain responsible for executive functions and self-regulation.

Improved attention is one of the most well-documented cognitive benefits of mindfulness. In a world filled with distractions, the ability to sustain focus is invaluable. Mindfulness practices train our attention to remain anchored in the present moment, helping us stay fully engaged in tasks and reducing mind-wandering and ruminative thinking.

Furthermore, mindfulness can enhance our capacity for self-awareness and self-reflection. By observing our thoughts and beliefs from a non-judgmental perspective, we gain insights into our mental patterns and can challenge unhelpful or negative thought patterns. This self-awareness is a cornerstone of personal growth and improved mental well-being.

Stress Reduction

Stress is a pervasive factor in modern life and a significant contributor to mental health challenges. Chronic stress can lead to a range of issues, including anxiety, depression, and burnout. Mindfulness offers a potent antidote to the negative effects of stress.

Through mindfulness practices, individuals can become more attuned to their stress triggers and responses. This heightened awareness allows them to respond to stressors more skillfully and make conscious choices to reduce their stress levels.

Mindfulness also promotes the relaxation response, which counteracts the stress response. Engaging in mindful activities like deep breathing or progressive muscle relaxation can induce a state of relaxation, lower cortisol levels (the stress hormone), and promote a sense of calm and equilibrium.

Building Resilience

Resilience is the capacity to bounce back from adversity and maintain psychological well-being in the face of life's challenges. Mindfulness plays a pivotal role in building resilience by fostering emotional flexibility and adaptability.

When we practice mindfulness, we learn to accept that life is inherently unpredictable and that difficulties are a natural part of the human experience. This acceptance does not imply resignation but rather a willingness to engage with life's challenges with an open heart and mind.

Mindfulness encourages us to view setbacks and failures as opportunities for growth rather than as insurmountable obstacles. This shift in perspective can empower individuals to develop resilience and navigate difficult circumstances with greater grace and fortitude.

Enhanced Self-Compassion

Self-compassion is the practice of treating oneself with the same kindness, understanding, and forgiveness that we would offer to a dear friend. It is a vital component of mental well-being, as it counteracts the self-criticism and negative self-talk that often contribute to emotional distress.

Mindfulness and self-compassion are intertwined. When we approach our inner experiences with mindfulness, we cultivate a non-judgmental and compassionate attitude towards ourselves. We learn to acknowledge our imperfections, vulnerabilities, and mistakes without self-condemnation.

This self-compassion can be a soothing balm for our mental well-being. It helps alleviate the burden of perfectionism and fosters a sense of self-worth and self-acceptance. When we treat ourselves with compassion, we are better equipped to weather life's challenges and maintain a positive self-image.

Improved Relationships

Our relationships with others are a significant factor in our mental well-being. Mindfulness can enhance the quality of our relationships by promoting empathy, active listening, and effective communication.

When we practice mindfulness, we become more present and attentive in our interactions with others. We listen with genuine interest and empathy, rather than simply waiting for our turn to speak. This deep listening fosters trust and intimacy in our relationships.

Additionally, mindfulness can reduce emotional reactivity in conflicts and disagreements. When we are mindful, we are less likely to react impulsively or defensively when faced with challenging situations. Instead, we can respond thoughtfully and empathetically, leading to more constructive and harmonious relationships.

Conclusion

In the pursuit of mental well-being, mindfulness emerges as a powerful and versatile tool. Its importance cannot be overstated, as it touches every aspect of our mental and emotional lives. By nurturing mindfulness practices, we can better regulate our emotions, enhance our cognitive abilities, reduce stress, build resilience, and foster self-compassion.

Mindfulness is not a panacea for all mental health challenges, but it provides us with a practical and accessible means to enhance our mental well-being. It equips us to navigate life's complexities with grace and resilience, ultimately leading to a more fulfilling and enriching life.

In the following chapters, we will delve

deeper into the practical aspects of mindfulness, exploring various techniques and exercises to help you incorporate mindfulness into your daily life. As you embark on this journey, remember that mindfulness is not a destination but a path—a path that leads to greater mental well-being, one mindful moment at a time.

1.3- Overview of the book's purpose and structure

Setting Out on a Conscious Transformation Journey

Here is where you may find "The Mindful Path: Navigating Mental Health Challenges with Resilience and Compassion." We cordially encourage you to set off on a life-changing adventure through the pages that follow, one that delves into the fundamental relationship between mental health and mindfulness. This book will accompany you on your journey across the complex terrain of your inner world, providing direction, understanding, and useful activities to improve your mental well-being and general quality of life.

This Book's Objective

The main goal of this book is to provide you the tools you need to take control of your mental health by using mindfulness's transformational power. This book is meant to give you the information, resources, and motivation you need, whether your goal is to fight depression, reduce stress and anxiety, or just improve your emotional resilience.

Our goal is not to provide quick cures or a one-size-fits-all solution. Rather, our goal is to enable you to develop mindfulness as a lifetime habit that permeates every aspect of your life and changes the way you see and react to the world. You can develop resilience, self-compassion, improve emotional control, and cultivate wholesome relationships by practising mindfulness.

Remember that every person has a different road to mental well-being as you set out on this adventure. You are solely responsible for your own experiences, difficulties, and goals. You can use this book as a roadmap to aid you on your own journey towards improved mental health.

The Book's Organisation

The framework of the book is crucial to understanding how to traverse this examination of mindfulness and mental health. Every chapter is meticulously constructed to expand upon the one before it, giving you a thorough grasp of the material along with useful activities and insights.

Chapter 1: Mindfulness's Significance for Mental Health

We explore the importance of mindfulness as the foundation of mental health in this first chapter. We look at the connections between the mind and body, emotional control, cognitive advantages, stress management, and the contribution of mindfulness to relationship improvement, resilience building, and self-compassion enhancement.

Chapter 2: Recognising Difficulties with Mental Health

It's important to know the terrain before starting any adventure. This chapter clarifies typical mental health issues, busts myths and false beliefs, and stresses the significance of getting help when you need it. Context and relatability are established through the weaving of personal tales and experiences.

Chapter 3: Mindfulness's Foundations

You need to grasp the fundamentals in order to lay a solid foundation. In Chapter 3, the fundamentals of mindfulness are presented, along with an explanation of what mindfulness is, its historical background, and the scientific data demonstrating its beneficial effects on mental health. Your mindfulness practise can be initiated with the use of useful exercises and techniques.

Chapter 4: Developing Hardiness

The capacity to overcome hardship is known as resilience, and it is an essential component of mental health. This chapter delves into the notion of resilience, the elements that influence it, and methods for developing increased resilience in one's life. Inspiration can be drawn from true accounts of those who have persevered in the face of adversity.

Chapter 5: Developing Compassion for Oneself

Despite being a fundamental component of mental health, self-compassion is frequently disregarded. This chapter walks you through the importance of self-compassion and how to develop it with mindfulness exercises. You'll discover how to accept and be kind to yourself in spite of your flaws and weaknesses.

Chapter 6: Relationships and Mindful Communication

Our mental health is greatly influenced by our connections. This chapter examines the ways in which mindfulness might improve our interpersonal relationships and communication. The value of creating supportive networks, mindful communication practises, and conflict resolution tactics are emphasised.

Chapter 7: Mindfulness and Stress Reduction

Stress is a common problem in our fast-paced society. Understanding the effects of stress on mental health and how mindfulness-based stress reduction practises can assist you in properly managing and mitigating stress are the main topics covered in Chapter 7. To reduce stress, we offer helpful advice on developing a mindful daily routine.

Chapter 8: Trauma Healing and Mindfulness

The effects of trauma can be significant on mental health. This chapter examines the many ways in which mindfulness might aid in the process of trauma recovery. It provides information on the relationship between trauma healing and mindfulness, as well as therapeutic strategies that integrate the two.

Chapter 9: Particular Populations' Mental Health and Mindfulness

Certain demographics may experience particular difficulties with mental health. In Chapter 9, it is discussed how mindfulness can be beneficially applied to children, teenagers, older adults, and people of different cultural backgrounds. It highlights how crucial cultural sensitivity is to mindfulness exercises.

Chapter 10: Maintaining a Mindful Path: Going Beyond the Book

As you draw closer to the end of this book, Chapter 10 offers advice on maintaining a mindful path after you leave these pages. It leaves you with parting thoughts on your mindful journey, options for continued support, and insights into integrating mindfulness into long-term mental health maintenance.Your Individual PathAs you proceed through the book's chapters, never forget that your path is entirely your own. You are welcome to go back over chapters that really speak to you, study the activities and strategies at your own speed, and modify the lessons to fit your particular requirements and situation.We urge you to practise patience and self-compassion on your journey. Developing mindfulness and improving mental health are ongoing processes rather than a final goal. It calls for effort, introspection, and a readiness to change and advance.

You are making a big step towards improved mental health by starting this journey with an open mind and an open heart. You're about to discover the life-changing potential of mindfulness, and the pages that follow are your roadmap to making it happen.

Chapter 2:
Challenges in Mental Health: A Better Understanding

2.1- Common mental health disorders (e.g., anxiety, depression, PTSD)

Title: Recognising and Coping with the Most Frequent Mental Health Conditions

Introduction

The state of one's mental health is crucial to their overall health and quality of life. However, just like with physical health, mental health can be negatively impacted by a wide range of ailments and disorders that manifest in a variety of ways. The purpose of this in-depth manual is to educate readers about common mental health issues like anxiety, sadness, and PTSD. To provide individuals and their loved ones with knowledge and resources to better understand and manage these issues, we will investigate the causes, symptoms, risk factors, and treatment choices for these disorders.

Anxiety: Navigating the Sea of Worry

Anxiety occurs as a normal reaction to pressure and is an integral component of being human. However, excessive and ongoing anxiety can develop into a diagnosable mental illness. Generalised Anxiety Disorder (GAD) is characterised by persistent and excessive concern over regular life occurrences. People with GAD have a hard time keeping their anxiety under control and may have physical symptoms like irritability, muscle tension, and trouble sleeping.

Depression: Fighting in Silence

One of the most common mental illnesses is depression. Depression is an extreme state of emotional distress that goes beyond simple feelings of sadness or gloom. No one is immune to the effects of Major Depressive Disorder (MDD), regardless of their age, gender, or socioeconomic status. Feelings of extreme melancholy, a lack of interest in formerly pleasurable activities, changes in eating and sleeping habits, extreme exhaustion, and even suicidal ideation are all symptoms of depression.

PTSD: Overcoming Adversity

Post-terrible Stress Disorder (PTSD) can occur after an individual encounters or observes a terrible event. Veterans of war, as well as those who have survived natural disasters or accidents, are not immune to this condition. Debilitating nightmares involving anxiety are not uncommon. However, debilitating dreams involving PTSD are. Recovery from post-traumatic stress disorder (PTSD) requires knowledge of both its causes and its treatments.

The Complicated Web of Influencing Factors

Mental health problems typically arise from a combination of variables including genetics, upbringing, and personality. Both external factors like trauma, abuse, or chronic stress, and a person's genetic susceptibility can contribute to the development of these diseases. The emergence of these disorders may also be aided by chemical abnormalities in the brain.

Understanding the Warning Signs

Early detection of mental health issues is crucial for quick management and improved outcomes. The following are examples of common symptoms:

1. an abnormally high level of persistent anxiety

2. extreme melancholy, or depression, characterised by a loss of interest in formerly pleasurable activities.
3 PTSD symptoms such as anxiety, flashbacks, and numbness.
Alterations in eating and sleeping habits
5. drained energy and weariness
Sixth, a lack of focus or indecision
Ability to have a mood fluctuation.
Eighth, retreat from social interaction
9. Physical complaints include headaches, stomachaches, or muscle strain
Ten. Suicidal or harm-inducing thoughts

Potential Dangers and Weaknesses

Some people are more likely to develop mental health problems because of their exposure to these risk factors. These include:

Symptoms of mental illness Symptoms of mental illness Symptoms of mental disease
2. Abuse or traumatic situations
3. Chronic stress 4. Substance abuse
5. Recurrent health problems
Sixth, chemical imbalances in the brain Seventh, major losses or changes in one's life
8. Loneliness and isolation

Seeking Assistance: Available Treatments

The good news is that there are effective treatments available for mental health problems. The first and most important step in dealing with these issues is to seek assistance from mental health specialists. Options for treatment may include:

1. Therapy: Psychotherapy, such as cognitive-behavioral therapy (CBT) or dialectical behaviour therapy (DBT), can help individuals

acquire coping techniques, detect thought patterns, and manage symptoms.

Second, Drugs: Medication is an option for treating symptoms in some situations. Common pharmaceuticals used to treat mental health issues include antidepressants, anti-anxiety drugs, and mood stabilisers.

Alterations to One's Way of Life Adopting a healthy lifestyle can have a profound effect on one's state of mind. Regular exercise, a balanced diet, proper sleep, and stress management strategies can all contribute to greater well-being.

Support Group Support Group Support Group Support Group Individuals can feel less alone and get a sense of community through participation in support groups or peer support.

Five Nonconventional Treatments: Alternative treatments such as yoga, acupuncture, and mindful meditation can be helpful for certain people.

Stigma and the Importance of Awareness

Despite the commonality of mental health problems, shame often stands in the way of people who could benefit from treatment. Those who suffer from these illnesses are generally misunderstood and shunned by mainstream society. The key to decreasing stigma and encouraging folks to seek the treatment they need without fear of judgement is to raise knowledge and promote understanding.

The Importance of Loved Ones

The help of loved ones cannot be overstated when it comes to coping with mental health issues. Lovers who learn more about these disorders are better able to understand and communicate with others who suffer from them. A person's support system can be bolstered by having family and friends participate in treatment or support groups with them.

The Road to Healing

Mental illness recovery is attainable. It's a long road that can have bumps in it, but with therapy and support, people can get their life back on track. It is crucial to recognise that healing is a personal process, and each individual's route is unique.

Conclusion

Improving the quality of life for those with mental health issues requires a better understanding of, and approach to, treatment. We can build a more caring and supporting community in which people may flourish in spite of the difficulties brought on by these conditions if we learn to see the warning signs, get the treatment they need, and spread the word. Never forget that your mental health is important and that you are not in this fight alone.

2.2- Stigma surrounding mental health

Speaking Out: The Fight Against Mental Health Stigma

Despite its importance to our well-being, mental health is still stigmatised, misunderstood, and little understood. The mental health stigma is engrained in our culture and has far-reaching effects on both individuals and groups. In this investigation, we will look into the persistent stigma that still plagues persons with mental health difficulties, investigate its roots, and talk about the crucial need of dispelling these preconceptions.

To paraphrase: The Roots of Stigma.

There has always been a stigma attached to discussing mental health. In the past, people with mental illness were often stigmatised and treated as though they were possessed or cursed because of their presumed connection to the supernatural. As a result of this false assumption, prejudice and discrimination persisted.

Stigma has remained over time despite our increased awareness of and ability to treat mental health conditions. This prejudice has many sources:

The belief that mental health disorders are a sign of personal weakness or a character flaw is pervasive, supporting the assumption that they are a sign of weakness or a flaw. These misunderstandings contribute to prejudice and isolation.

2. The Power of the Media: Misconceptions about people with mental health issues have been spread widely thanks to the media and entertainment industry. This furthers the stigmatisation of mental health issues when characters with them are portrayed as dangerous, unstable, or untreatable.

Thirdly, Social and Cultural Beliefs: The stigma attached to mental health may have roots in cultural and societal expectations. Seeking mental health care may be seen as a sign of weakness or embarrassment in some cultures.

Aversion to the Unknown (4) Stigma can also be caused by the unknown inducing feelings of fear and discomfort. Some people don't realise how common mental health issues are or that anyone can be affected by them.

The Repercussions of Social Shame

Negative attitudes towards mental health can have far-reaching and serious repercussions.

Impediments to Treatment 1. When people feel ashamed, they are less likely to ask for assistance. People may be hesitant to seek help from mental health specialists due to concerns about stigma.

2. Delayed Diagnosis: Many people may be undiagnosed or untreated for long periods of time due to the reluctance to seek treatment. Their diseases may worsen and their symptoms may become more severe as a result of this delay.

Felt alienation and isolation (3): Isolation is a potential outcome of stigmatising sentiments. People with mental health issues may isolate themselves for fear of stigma or rejection.

Self-Stigma, number 4. Self-stigma occurs when an individual internalises negative social stereotypes about themselves. Such a view of oneself can be a major roadblock to healing.

5. Relationship Impact: Relationships with loved ones, friends, and coworkers can all be negatively impacted by stigma. Some people

may avoid interacting with those who are struggling with mental health because they fear being judged.

The Importance of Raise[ing] People's Aware[ness]

Education and advocacy are crucial in the fight against the stigma associated with mental health issues. Stereotypes and prejudice are difficult to overcome, but efforts to increase comprehension and compassion can help. Some essential tactics are as follows:

1. Frank Discussions: When people are able to talk freely about their struggles with mental health, it fosters a supportive community. These discussions can help bring the issues home to people and debunk falsehoods.

2. Media Accountability: The media has a great deal of sway over how people feel about things. Stigma can be reduced with the help of accurate depictions of mental health in media including movies, TV shows, and news reporting.

Education Programmes : Education Programmes : Education Programme By introducing programmes on mental health to classrooms and workplaces, people can gain access to reliable resources on the subject. Empathy is a byproduct of comprehension.

Four, Stories: Success stories from people who have dealt with mental health issues and the associated stigma are potent agents of change. One can gain hope and strength from reading these accounts.

5. Available Materials Making available readily available tools and services in the field of mental health can promote early intervention and treatment. Making it easier for people to get aid is essential.

Promoting Kindness as a Core Value

Last but not least, we need a cultural shift towards compassion and understanding in order to successfully battle mental health stigma. Stigmatising sentiments sometimes come from fear and misinformation. We can create an atmosphere where people feel secure and encouraged in seeking help when they need it by cultivating a society that values mental health as much as physical health and by encouraging open discourse.

Self-Stigma and How to Get Past It

Self-stigma needs to be addressed at the same time as societal stigma. It's common for people with mental health issues to internalise blame and have negative ideas about their conditions. To get past self-stigmatization:

First, it's important to educate yourself on your mental health condition and its therapy. Realising that mental health problems are physical conditions rather than moral failings can have a profound effect on one's outlook.

[2] Self-Compassion: Combating self-stigma requires regular practise of self-compassion and self-acceptance. Keep in mind that one's mental health does not indicate their value or character.

3. Peer Support: Sharing your struggles with others who understand is a great way to gain acceptance and encouragement. When it comes to overcoming internalised stigma, peer support groups might be helpful.

4. Professional treatment: Seeking treatment from mental health specialists is vital. They can help with diagnosis, treatment, and overcoming internalised stigma.

Getting Past Stigma and Into the Future

Overcoming the stigma around mental health is an ongoing process that involves the joint work of individuals, communities, and society at large. It starts with realising that mental health is an intrinsic element of total well-being and that mental health disorders are not a sign of weakness or failure.

We can make the world a better place for people struggling with their mental health by spreading awareness, compassion, and honest discussion. If we work together, we can end the stigma around mental health and pave the path for it to be regarded with the same respect as physical health in the future.

2.3- Personal stories and experiences

Advocacy in the Field of Mental Health: The Impact of Personal Stories

Personal narratives and experiences are powerful catalysts for change, sources of empathy, and busters of myths in the field of mental health advocacy and awareness. These first-person accounts by those who have struggled with mental health issues shed light on a field that is often difficult to discuss openly. We will examine how telling one's own story can help break down barriers of stigma, increase comprehension, and inspire optimism in the realm of mental health activism.

An Insight into the Human Condition

One way to understand the complexity of mental health is through people's own tales. They go beyond dry data and clinical descriptions to let us empathise with actual people and their experiences. When someone opens up about their experience with mental health issues, it helps normalise and reduce the stigma of talking about it.

There are several possible structures for such tales:

- Survivor Stories: People who have struggled with mental health but have found healing share their experiences.

Narratives of people's lives and the ways in which they've dealt with the stresses of modern-day life and the challenges of coping with the realities of their own and others' mental health issues.

- Carer Perspectives: loved ones and friends of people with mental illness share their experiences as carers to shed light on the difficulties experienced by everyone involved.

Dispelling Prejudice

One of the most major barriers to receiving care for mental health disorders is stigma. Stigma is caused by preconceived notions and ignorance, and it often results in people suffering in silence. Stories from real people are crucial in combating these harmful stereotypes.

When people share their stories, when they:

1. Humanise the Experience: First-hand accounts show that anyone of any age, gender, or socioeconomic status can suffer from mental health problems. This destigmatization reduces the stigma associated with mental health by making it seem less "other."

To Challenge Stereotypes, tell tales from your own life that directly contradict common beliefs. Examples of high-functioning people who manage their mental illness despite this stigma are one way this myth might be disproved.

Encourage Compassion: Hearing about someone's story might create empathy and understanding in others. It helps people empathise with persons who are experiencing mental health issues by putting themselves in their position.

To people who are currently going through a difficult time, stories of triumph over adversity offer hope. Those who are feeling hopeless may find solace in hearing how others have triumphed over adversity.

Make asking for assistance the norm Seeking aid and getting treatment are common themes in personal narratives. These accounts urge others to seek assistance by showing that doing so is commonplace.

Reducing the Stigma of Mental Health Issues.

The stigma surrounding many mental health issues dates back millennia. Misconceptions and prejudice exist towards people with mental health issues such as depression, anxiety, bipolar illness, and schizophrenia. Telling one's own story about overcoming the stigma associated with these illnesses can be quite effective.

Understanding the crippling impact of depression and anxiety is made easier by hearing first-hand accounts from others who have overcome it. They stress the value of treatment and provide advice on how to manage symptoms.

Bipolar Disorder: Personal accounts from those living with bipolar disorder help dispel myths about their mood swings and show how productive and happy life can be when the disorder is properly managed.

Schizophrenia: Personal accounts of coping with schizophrenia disprove the stereotype that people with the disorder are dangerous and irrational. The importance of early intervention and social support structures is emphasised.

Individual experiences with anorexia and bulimia provide light on the intricacies of these diseases and the elements that contribute to their development and the road to recovery.

Survivors of post-traumatic stress disorder (PTSD) share their experiences in order to shed light on the effects of trauma and the value of trauma-informed care.

There is safety in numbers when sharing experiences.

Individuals foster a more supportive and accepting environment by discussing their experiences with mental health. The realisation that others have endured similar problems might decrease the isolation that often accompanies mental health conditions. Having a group of people who "get you" is a tremendous source of strength and perseverance.

The benefits of social interaction extend beyond the alleviation of loneliness.

- Stimulate Seeking Assistance Knowing that others have sought help and benefited from it can encourage those who are struggling to do the same.

- Suggest Ways to Deal With Stress Personal narratives frequently reveal the narrator's successful methods of dealing with adversity. Those who are experiencing similar difficulties may find these methods extremely helpful.

Create a System of Support: The establishment of peer groups and support networks is facilitated by the sharing of experiences. These online communities facilitate communication and the exchange of useful information among members.

The Culture of Exposure

Being open and honest about one's own struggles with mental health is important. To be vulnerable is to share one's innermost thoughts and feelings in a public setting. It takes bravery to be this open, but doing so is crucial to normalising discussions about mental health.

When folks are willing to be vulnerable and share their stories:

First, by opening up about their own struggles with mental health, those who do so encourage others to do the same.

They break the hush in the second verse. Silence has long been associated with a stigma against mental health. Sharing one's own experiences is a great way to break the ice and start a conversation.

Thirdly, they promote being one's true self. Personal experiences increase honesty in discussions about mental health. Sincerity is the seed from which understanding and friendship grow.

They are great conversation starters; Sharing one's life experiences is a common way to start conversations with neighbours and acquaintances. These discussions have the potential to dramatically impact efforts to reduce stigma.

The Impact on Policy and Healthcare

Personal experiences have the potential to affect healthcare policy and practise at the systemic level. Hearing these stories can help politicians, healthcare practitioners, and other organisations better understand the realities of living with a mental health issue. This knowledge can be used to better allocate resources and advocate for those in need of mental health care.

Finishing Thoughts and Feelings

Personal narratives are incredibly important in the continuous effort to remove the stigma associated with mental health. They can inspire hope in the hopeless, alter people's perspectives, and break through barriers of prejudice. People who have struggled with mental health can help others and make the world a better place just by opening up and talking about their experiences. A future where mental health is treated with the same acceptance and support as any other health condition is one step closer with every story told.

Chapter 3:
What You Need to Know About Mindfulness

3.1- What is mindfulness?

Getting to the Heart of Mindfulness

In a fast-paced society packed with distractions and pressures, mindfulness has evolved as a profound practise that brings calm, clarity, and a deeper connection to the present moment. Mindfulness has attracted the interest of individuals, scientists, and practitioners because it is more than just a catchphrase; it is a truly transformational way of life. We will examine the meaning of mindfulness, where it came from, how it might improve our lives, and what it takes to make it a regular part of our routine.

Mindfulness: A Definition

Mindfulness, in its essence, is the practise of living in the here and now with openness, curiosity, and acceptance rather than resistance or judgement. Paradigms of old and current wisdom are entwined in our practise.

Mindfulness is "the awareness that arises through paying attention, on purpose, in the present moment, nonjudgmentally," as described by Jon Kabat-Zinn, a leader in popularising mindfulness in the West. Intention, presence, and nonjudgment are all covered by this definition of mindfulness.

Roots of Being Present

The practise of mindfulness has ancient roots in many religions and philosophies. It is commonly used in Buddhist meditation and has become synonymous with the religion. Mindfulness, or "sati" in Pali and "smti" in Sanskrit, is a practise that has been developed over the course of more than two thousand five hundred years.

Sati means giving conscious attention to one's ideas, feelings, body sensations, and surroundings without attachment or aversion. Its goal is to help people get perspective and realise that everything is fleeting.

The Recent Mindfulness Trend

While mindfulness has ancient beginnings, its present appeal may be traced back to the late 20th century. The Mindfulness-Based Stress Reduction (MBSR) programme was established in 1979 by medical professor Jon Kabat-Zinn at the University of Massachusetts Medical School. This show reworked mindfulness techniques for a nonreligious audience, highlighting their ability to lessen anxiety and boost well-being.

Mindfulness has since entered the mainstream, making its way into fields as diverse as medicine, psychology, education, and the workplace. To address a wide range of mental and physical health issues, including anxiety, depression, chronic pain, and addiction, mindfulness-based interventions (MBIs) have been created.

What It's Like to Practise Mindfulness

Mindfulness encourages us to turn off the automatic pilot of our hectic lives and instead pay closer attention to the internal and external experiences that make up our life. Some essential parts of a mindful experience are as follows:

1. Being Aware of the Present With the help of mindfulness, we can stop thinking about the past or the future and instead focus on what's happening right now. Focusing one's attention on the here and now is a deliberate act.

1. Observation: n. 1. N. J. Observation: n. Without passing judgement on our thoughts and actions, we cannot fully practise mindfulness. This involves paying attention to one's internal experiences as they occur, without assigning value judgements.

3. Self-Compassion and Acceptance: Mindfulness encourages both. It encourages us to be gentle with ourselves, since we are all flawed humans.

4. Using Breath as a Foundation In mindful meditation, the breath is frequently employed as a focal point. To bring one's attention back to the present moment when the mind wanders, focusing on the breath is a tried and true method.

5. Refining the Art of Silence Stillness, as in seated meditation, and movement, as in mindful walking or yoga, are both valid ways to cultivate mindfulness. Both techniques emphasise a purposeful and focused attentiveness.

The Value of Being Present

Extensive research into the practise of mindfulness has revealed numerous physiological, psychological, and emotional advantages, including the following.

Reducing stress and its symptoms is one of the primary goals of mindfulness-based therapies. The negative consequences of prolonged stress can be reduced through the mindful recognition of stressors and the application of nonreactive coping mechanisms.

2. Better Emotional Regulation: Being mindful helps you become more in tune with and in control of your feelings. It lets individuals to examine their emotions without quickly reacting to them, enabling space to choose more balanced answers.

Increased Capacity for Concentration and Focus: Consistent mindfulness practise has been shown to increase focus and attention, making it less taxing to maintain attention on a task over the long term.

4. More Restful Nights Reduce rumination and sleep better with the help of mindfulness techniques.

5. Pain Management: Mindfulness-based treatments have demonstrated potential in alleviating pain and enhancing the quality of life for people living with chronic pain.

6. Improved Happiness: Mindfulness training has been linked to higher levels of happiness and fulfilment in one's life.

7. Reduced Symptoms of Anxiety and Depression: Mindfulness-based therapies have been shown beneficial in reducing symptoms of anxiety and depression, giving an alternative or supplementary approach to treatment.

Enhanced Connections, Number Eight By making one more aware of and attuned to the feelings and needs of those around them, mindfulness can improve communication, empathy, and emotional connection in interpersonal interactions.

Practising Everyday Mindfulness

Its beauty lies in its simplicity and its versatility. The positive effects of meditation can be felt in as little as ten minutes a day. Here are some easy methods to practise mindfulness every day:

Mindful breathing is the first technique. Take a few moments each day to focus on your breath. Try closing your eyes as you take a few calm, deep breaths in through your nose and out through your mouth. Focus on the feeling of air going in and out of your lungs.

Conscious Eating Eat slowly and savour every bite. Think on how each dish looks, tastes, and feels as you eat it. Take your time chewing and enjoy the food you're eating.

Body scan 3: Scan your body before bed or when you first get up. Focus on your toes, then work your way up your body, taking note of any places of stress or pain along the way.

4. Mindful Walking: Pay attention to each stride you take while walking. Take awareness of your body's motion and the environment around you by feeling the floor with your feet.

Pause for Reflection 5. Pause for reflection periodically during the day. Put an end to your current activity, take a few deep breaths, and bring your attention back to the here and now.

6. Conscious Technological Habitat: Give thought to how you use technology. Put down the screen every once in a while and bring your whole attention to whatever you're doing.

7. Exercises in Gratitude: Practise daily gratitude by thinking about three things you're thankful for. Focusing on the good things in your life is the goal of this exercise.

Final Thoughts on "The Priceless Present"

A road to deeper self-awareness, inner calm, and well-being, mindfulness is a priceless gift. It serves as a timely reminder that our lives are more than just a collection of chores and errands; they are also a sequence of priceless moments deserving of our undivided attention. Mindfulness is a powerful tool for cultivating meaningful relationships with oneself, others, and the world at large.

3.2- Benefits of mindfulness for mental health

Meditation Improves Emotional and Mental Health

The value of taking care of your mental health in today's fast-paced, high-stress society cannot be stressed. Anxiety, sadness, and other mental health problems are common when the responsibilities of job, family, and personal life become too much to bear. Thankfully, there is a wide range of methods and practises available to assist with mental health management. Mindfulness is one such practise that has exploded in popularity in recent years.

The practise of mindfulness, which has its origins in Eastern philosophy but has been modified for contemporary use, is a potent method of improving one's emotional and physical health. Being mindful means paying attention to the here and now without judgement. This technique teaches people to be impartial observers of their inner experiences, including emotions and body sensations. Beyond the mere act of being present, the advantages of meditation go well beyond the realm of the mind.

In this piece, we will delve into the many advantages of mindfulness for the mind, demonstrating its transforming potential for people who want to boost their emotional health and live a more well-rounded existence.

1. Reducing Stress

One of the most commonly recognised benefits of mindfulness is its capacity to relieve stress. Today's hectic lifestyles are a major contributor to the widespread epidemic of chronic stress that has negative effects on both physical and mental health. Mindfulness helps individuals become more aware of their stressors and reactions, helping them to respond to stressful situations with better serenity and resilience. Regular practise of mindfulness has been shown to reduce cortisol, the body's primary stress hormone, and, in turn, the effects of stress.

Controlling Your Worries

Constant worry and fear can be debilitating, and millions of individuals worldwide suffer from anxiety disorders. Evidence suggests that practising mindfulness can help people with anxiety. Being more aware of one's anxious thoughts and sensations in the body through mindfulness practises can help one stop dwelling on them and calm down. Anxious sensations can be mitigated by concentrating on the here and now and practising deep breathing techniques.

Increased Capacity to Control Emotions

Being mindful helps you become more self-aware and in control of your emotions. It teaches people to accept their feelings as neutral experiences that come and go with time. The ability to maintain one's composure in the face of strong emotions can be greatly enhanced by adopting a non-reactive stance. Mindfulness can help people become more emotionally resilient and improve their emotional reactions over time.

Increased Insight into Oneself

Self-awareness is crucial to one's psychological well-being and development. The practise of mindfulness encourages introspection and awareness of one's inner processes. Mindfulness training helps people learn more about themselves, their beliefs, and their actions. This improved self-awareness can lead to better self-acceptance and personal growth.

Fifthly, it helps with focus and concentration.

Many people find it difficult to concentrate and focus in today's chaotic society. Mindfulness improves mental performance by teaching people to pay attention in the here and now. Practises like deep breathing and body scanning can help improve focus and concentration, leading to greater efficiency in all areas of life.

6. High-Quality Sleep

Many people suffer from sleep disorders or chronic insomnia, despite the importance of sleep to mental health. There is evidence that interventions focused on mindfulness can help people get a better night's sleep by calming the mind and relieving stress. Relaxation techniques like meditation and progressive muscle relaxation can help people get to sleep more quickly and more easily.

7 Depressive Symptoms are Lessened

Complex and incapacitating, depression is a serious mental illness. While mindfulness is not a replacement for professional treatment, it can be a beneficial adjunct to therapy and medicine. The purpose of mindfulness-based cognitive therapy (MBCT) is to help people who suffer from depression avoid falling back into their old patterns. MBCT can lessen the frequency of depression episodes by helping people learn to spot their symptoms early and respond with mindfulness practises.

Gains in Resistance to Stress

The capacity to recover quickly from setbacks and successfully navigate difficult circumstances is what we mean when we talk about resilience. Through cultivating equanimity in the face of adversity, mindfulness helps people persevere. Mindfulness training helps people bounce back from challenges and hardships, strengthening their resilience.

Nine. Better Connections

Positive effects of mindfulness on relationships are also supported by research. Better listening and communicating skills develop when people are able to focus on the current moment and pay closer attention to their internal experiences. They are less inclined to respond hastily or defensively, creating better and more compassionate connections with others. As a result, you should expect to see improvements in your relationships at home and at work.

Ten. Increased Happiness and Contentment

In the end, practising mindfulness can help you feel better about life in general. It encourages people to stop pining for a better tomorrow and start appreciating what they have right now. Those who are able to let go of their preoccupation with the past and the future are better able to enjoy the present moment.

Ultimately, the benefits of mindfulness to one's mental health are far too many to ignore. It is a useful tool for people who want to better their mental health and lead more satisfying lives because of its ability to alleviate stress, control anxiety, increase emotional regulation, heighten self-awareness, strengthen focus, enhance sleep quality, decrease depressive symptoms, fortify resilience, strengthen relationships, and promote happiness.

Mindfulness can be practised on its own, but it can also be included into other forms of therapy and treatment for psychological issues. Mindfulness has been shown to have positive effects on mental health and wellbeing, and can be practised on its own or as part of a larger therapy programme. If you haven't already, start practising mindfulness every day to reap the life-changing mental health advantages it has to offer.

3.3- Practical exercises and techniques

Meditation and other Mindful Practises.

Now that we've covered the many ways in which mindfulness can improve your mental health, we'll look at some exercises and strategies for incorporating mindfulness into your daily life. These routines are made to be flexible so that you can modify them to fit your own needs. Mindfulness is a skill that can be honed with consistent practise, so remember to be kind with yourself.

(1) Concentrated breathing:

One of the most basic and accessible forms of mindfulness practise is paying attention to one's breathing. You simply observe your breathing without interfering with it in any way. This is the procedure:

   - Go somewhere you can relax in peace and quiet.
   - If it makes you feel more at ease, close your eyes and take a few deep breaths.
   - Focus on your breathing for a moment. Notice the sensation of the breath entering and leaving your nostrils or the rise and fall of your chest or abdomen.
   - Focus on your breathing by telling yourself, "I am breathing in." As you breathe out, say, "I am breathing out." Keep doing this, using the breath as a focal point for your awareness.

When your thoughts wander, return them to the breath without criticism. Start with a short session each day and build up to longer ones as you gain experience.

2. Mindful Body Scan:

Part of being present in the moment is being aware of where your attention is going as you move through your day. It helps you become more aware of physical sensations and can be particularly effective for relieving tension and stress. This is the procedure:

Get yourself to a nice, quiet spot, and take a nap.
- Take a few deep breaths and close your eyes to relax.
- Start from the tips of your toes and work your way up, focusing on each part of your body in turn and noting any tightness or unusual feelings as you go.
- Try to let go of whatever stress you feel as you go along. If your shoulders are tense, for instance, try intentionally unwinding them as you exhale.
- To complete a full body scan, just keep going.

When done at evening, a body scan can be a wonderful way to wind down and unwind.

Meditation while walking

The act of walking mindfully is a technique to incorporate mindfulness into your daily routine. This workout can be done anywhere, whether you're strolling through a park, your neighbourhood, or your own living room. How to train your mind to walk mindfully:

To get yourself in the right frame of mind, stop what you're doing and take a few deep breaths.
Focus on the feeling of your feet leaving the ground, flying through the air, and touching down on the surface with each stride as you start to walk.
- Focus on the sensations of walking, including the earth beneath your feet and the cadence of your steps.
- If you find your thoughts wandering, gently draw them back to the act of walking itself.

Walking with awareness can help you tune in to your surroundings and free your thoughts of clutter.

4. Eating With Purpose:

By bringing your complete attention to the act of eating, you practise mindful eating. Overeating may be avoided, and you can learn to have a healthier relationship with food. To eat more mindfully, try these steps:

   Pick a bite-sized serving of your favourite cuisine.
   - Take a seat at the table and savour the taste, aroma, and texture of your meal.
   - As you chew, pay attention to the tastes, smells, and textures that come to light as you chew. Take your time chewing and enjoy every bite.
   - Avoid multitasking while eating by ignoring your phone or turning off the TV.

When you eat with awareness, you learn to recognise when you're full and stop eating before you feel sick.

5. Meditation on Loving-Kindness:

Loving-kindness Metta meditation is a form of mindfulness in which the practitioner sends loving thoughts and intentions to themselves and others. It may help people feel more connected and compassionate. This is the procedure:

   - Go somewhere you can relax in peace and quiet.
   - Put your focus inward, and close your eyes.
   Start by sending warm thoughts and feelings to yourself. Sayings like "May I be happy" should be repeated. I pray for good health. I pray for a life of ease.

- After waiting a short while, turn your attention to a loved one and share these sentiments with them.
- As you go on, remember to be compassionate not just to those you know well but also to those with whom you may have disagreements and, finally, to all beings.

Loving-kindness meditation can develop feelings of empathy and connection with others while fostering self-compassion.

Incorporating mindfulness into your daily life is easier than you think with the help of these simple exercises and practises. Try out many methods until you find one that clicks with you. Mindfulness has the potential to become an essential component of your mental health toolkit, equipping you to face life's obstacles with increased fortitude, self-awareness, and overall well-being. To fully experience the positive effects of mindfulness on your mental health, remember that persistence and perseverance are essential.

Chapter 4:
Strengthening Resistance

4.1- Resilience as a key factor in mental health

The Crucial Role of Resilience in Psychological Health

When we are emotionally, psychologically, and socially well, we are said to be in good mental health. This state of affairs is a result of a combination of genetics, environment, life events, and personal coping methods, and it can change over time. Resilience is a distinguishing feature within the intricate web of mental health and a potent predictor of success in life.

The ability to recover quickly from setbacks and successfully adjust to new circumstances—qualities commonly referred to as "resilience"—are crucial for preserving and fostering sound mental health. Being able to deal with the ups and downs of life requires not only a lack of mental disease but also a solid psychological foundation. The importance of resilience to mental health and methods for fostering it will be discussed in this article.

How to Build Resistance to Stress

Rather than being an immutable characteristic, resilience is a process that can be developed and honed through time. Resilience is the ability to bounce back from failures, continue pushing forward, and ultimately succeeding despite the odds. People who are resilient are not impervious to stress, trauma, or adversity; rather, they have developed coping mechanisms that make it easier for them to deal with adversity.

Key Components of Resilience:

Resilient people have mastered the art of emotional regulation, or the ability to both identify and control their feelings. They are able to deal with their emotions rationally, without stuffing them down or denying their existence.

2. Adaptability: Resilience is tied to the capacity to modify one's objectives and methods of operation in response to adversity. To be resilient, one must be able to think and act creatively in the face of adversity.

(3) Social Support: Resilience requires a solid group of friends and family to lean on in times of need. In trying circumstances, it helps immensely to have people around who care enough to offer both emotional and practical support.

4. Optimism and Positive Outlook: People who are able to bounce back from adversity do so because they are able to keep their sense of optimism and hope despite their circumstances. They have faith in their own resiliency and view setbacks as transient.
5. Self-Confidence: Belief in one's own capabilities is crucial to bouncing back from adversity. It empowers people to face hardship with a sense of strength and determination.
Having a variety of problem-solving, seeking-help, self-care, and meaning-finding coping skills at your disposal is an important part of being resilient.

The Importance of Resilience to One's Emotional Well-Being

One of resilience's primary functions is to mitigate stress's potentially harmful effects. Anxiety and depression are two examples of mental health conditions that can be exacerbated by stress. Those who are more resilient are better able to deal with and lessen the effects of stress on their mental health.

Second, resilience can be used as a preventative measure to lessen the likelihood that one will experience mental health problems later in life. When individuals have good coping mechanisms and emotional regulation skills, they are less sensitive to the adverse impacts of life's obstacles.

Resilience is essential in the healing process for people who have suffered from mental health problems or traumatic experiences. It helps people recover their sense of purpose and well-being after experiencing trauma and aids in their healing process.
Those who are able to bounce back from adversity more quickly tend to be happier and more fulfilled with life. They have greater resilience and an optimistic outlook, both of which contribute to an improved quality of life.

Effective Methods to Improve Your Capacity to Bounce Back
1. Cultivate Social Connections: Create and sustain meaningful relationships with loved ones and people in your community who have your back. Adversarial situations are made easier by the emotional support provided by these partnerships.

Work on your Emotional Intelligence by learning to recognise and control your feelings. Mindfulness and meditation are two practises that have been shown to help in emotional control.

Third, Set Realistic Goals: Create objectives that can be attained with some effort and be willing to change them as circumstances demand. When faced with adversity, this prevents a sense of failure or disappointment.

Fourth, practise Positive Self-Talk by rebutting critical self-talk with compassion optimism. Treat yourself kindly and concentrate on your virtues.

5. Practise Creative Problem Solving Improve your ability to solve problems by learning to break them down into smaller, more manageable chunks. Instead of getting discouraged, try to find ways around the problem.

6. Practise Mindfulness: Activities like meditation and deep breathing are great examples of mindfulness practises that can help you stay in the present and less anxious about the future.
If you are experiencing mental health problems, it is important that you seek the assistance of a trained professional. The skills and encouragement gained through therapy are invaluable resources for building fortitude.

Put yourself first and make self-care a regular part of your schedule. Sleeping enough, eating right, being physically active, and doing things that you enjoy are all important components of a healthy lifestyle.

Opportunity in adversity: Learn to see failures as learning opportunities, not as setbacks. Think about what you've learned from adversity.

Tenth, make gratitude a habit by consistently reflecting on and celebrating the good things in your life. This may enable you to adopt a more optimistic mindset.

11. Perform Acts of Kindness: Doing good deeds for other people can make you feel good about yourself and strengthen your relationships, both of which are important components of resilience.

Create a positive atmosphere by surrounding oneself with positive, encouraging people. Get away from or reduce your time spent in harmful situations.

Building Resilience Into Your Routine

Resilience is developed through a series of daily decisions and routines. Strengthening your resilience and enhancing your mental health is not an overnight process, but it is possible with hard work and dedication. Here are some suggestions for practising resilience every day:

1. Morning Reflection: Take a few moments each morning to think about the day ahead. Determine that you will face adversity with optimism and strength.

2. Mindful Moments: Take frequent, brief opportunities to pause and focus on the present moment. Take a few slow, deep breaths to centre yourself.

3. Connect with Support: Reach out to friends or family members when you need support or simply to connect. The process of establishing a network of allies is never-ending.

4. Maintain a Resilience Journal: The concept of "resilience" is a bit of a mis Keep a notebook in which you detail your experiences with resiliency, the challenges you've faced, and the ways in which you've conquered them. Having this might give you hope when things seem hopeless.

5. Self-Care Rituals: Make time in your schedule for self-care activities like yoga in the morning, a walk before bed, or a monthly spa day. Taking care of yourself in these ways strengthens your mental fortitude.

6. Take Inspiration from Role Models: Look for and study the lives of people who have overcome adversity. Their words and deeds can serve as a source of wisdom and motivation for others.

Regardless of how insignificant you may think your successes are, it is important to recognise and honour them. Confidence and resilience can be boosted by taking stock of one's accomplishments.

Final Reflections

Rather than being a static quality, resilience is a skill that can be developed and honed over time. It's crucial to mental health because it helps people cope with stress, stops them from developing mental health problems, and speeds up their recovery after experiencing trauma. Individuals can handle life's difficulties better if they adopt methods and routines that boost resilience.

and continue to have a healthy mental state.

Keep in mind that developing resilience is a process that will need time and kindness towards yourself. It's about providing oneself with the tools and mindsets necessary to tackle hardship with courage and positivity. In the process of taking this journey, you will learn how the trait of resilience may have a profound effect on your mental health for the better.

4.2- Strategies for developing resilience

Methods for Building Resistance

Individuals that possess the quality of resilience are able to overcome setbacks, remain flexible in the face of change, and prosper regardless of the circumstances they find themselves in. It's not something you're born with; rather, it's a collection of faculties you develop and hone over time. Building resilience is important for people's emotional well-being because it improves their ability to deal with stress, adversity, and other challenging life events. In this post, we will cover a range of practical ideas and practises that can help individuals develop and strengthen their resilience.

Develop a "growth mindset"

The idea that one's strengths and intelligence may be cultivated via hard work and study is central to the "growth mindset." Adopting a "growth mindset" has been shown to increase resilience considerably. Setbacks are less intimidating when seen through the lens of learning and development possibilities. You don't view setbacks as fatal; rather, you use them as learning opportunities. To foster a growth perspective, one must:

Rather than shying away from difficulty, embrace it as a chance to learn and grow.
Recast setbacks as instructive lessons.
Pay more attention to the steps you're doing to get better than of the results you're hoping to achieve.

The second piece of advice is to work on your EQ.

Being able to identify, analyse, and control one's own emotions as well as those of others is a hallmark of emotional intelligence. It's a vital part of being resilient since it makes it easier to deal with challenging events and maintain positive connections. In order to develop your emotional quotient:

Check in with your feelings and figure out what sets them off; this is a form of self-awareness.
Develop your capacity for empathy by making an effort to put yourself in the shoes of others around you.
Relaxation exercises, mindful awareness, and other positive coping strategies can all help you gain control over your feelings.

3. Establish Solid Friendships

Resilience is greatly enhanced by the presence of social support. Having a solid network of friends, family, and community members to fall back on during hard times is invaluable. Paraphrase To strengthen your social contacts.

- Prioritise spending time with loved ones and strengthening your relationships.
- Reach out for support when required and be willing to offer support to others.
- Get involved with communities that share your interests and values.

4. Learn to Solve Problems

One of the cornerstones of resilience is the ability to effectively solve problems. It gives you the ability to deliberately approach problems, reduce them to more manageable chunks, and solve them. In order to learn how to solve problems,

Get specific when describing the issue.
Create a wide range of options, even if some of them are out of the ordinary.
Weigh the benefits of each option and choose on the best course of action.

- Do something, keep an eye on the results, and change tactics if necessary.

Fifthly, "Be Mindful" and "Take Care of Yourself"

Being mindful means paying attention to the present without passing judgement on it. It can aid in stress management, anxiety reduction, and improved control over one's emotions. Incorporating mindfulness practises into your everyday routine can contribute to resilience. Here are some practises to try to cultivate more awareness:

- Mindful Breathing: Dedicate some time every day to paying attention to, but not altering, your breathing pattern. Doing so can aid in relaxing the mind and body.

To become attuned to bodily sensations and alleviate muscular tension, try using a body scan meditation.

- Mindful Walking: Practise mindful walking by focusing on each step and the physical sensations of walking.

- Daily Gratitude: Make it a routine to think about and be thankful for the good things in your life. A more optimistic view and greater fortitude can result from this.

Include self-care rituals—like physical activity, meditation, reading, and time in nature—in your daily schedule.

6. Plan Ahead with Reasonable Objectives

By avoiding the negative emotions associated with failure and disappointment, which can weaken resilience, setting and maintaining realistic objectives and expectations is essential. In order to aim appropriately:

Reduce overwhelming tasks into more manageable chunks.
Keep an open mind and be willing to adjust your plans if necessary.
- Rejoice in your successes, no matter how insignificant they may appear at the time.

7 Get Expert Help If You Need It

Courageous people don't have to take on adversity on their own. The most courageous move you can do in such a situation may be to consult a trained therapist or counsellor. Counsellors and psychotherapists are available to help people deal with their emotional distress and the effects of traumatic events.

8. Gain Wisdom from Adversity

Challenges and failures can teach us invaluable lessons. Think of setbacks not as something to be avoided at all costs but as challenges to be overcome and lessons to be learned. Ponder these

What am I supposed to take out from this?
How have I grown as a person as a result of this difficulty?
How can I use this knowledge in the future?

9. Practise Self-Compassion

To practise self-compassion, you need to be as patient and forgiving with yourself as you would be with a close friend. Managing one's own stoicism and positive self-image is a critical element of any successful business. Compassion for oneself entails:

Negative self-talk and self-criticism should be avoided at all costs.
- Treat yourself with the same warmth and empathy you would show to a loved one.
- Keep in mind that you're human, thus you're allowed to make errors and struggle.

Ten. Remain Adaptable and Flexible

Being able to modify one's objectives and approach as necessary is a key component of resilience. When things don't go as planned, rigidity can cause a person to feel hopeless and frustrated. Maintain a growth mindset and an adaptable strategy.

11. Acts of Kindness,

One of the best ways to strengthen your own resilience is to help others through acts of kindness. As an added bonus, assisting others is a great way to take your mind off of your own problems.

12 Keep a Journal of Resilience

Keeping a journal is a great way to practise mindfulness, which has been shown to increase resilience. In your journal, document your experiences of resilience, problems you've conquered, and the techniques that worked for you. Keep this journal close to remind you of your inner power and use it as a source of motivation whenever you need it.

Celebrate the Little Victories

Recognising and appreciating your successes, no matter how seemingly insignificant, helps strengthen your self-esteem and fortitude. Don't forget to celebrate your successes and acknowledge your tenacity in the face of adversity.

BuildSupportiveEnvironment

Put yourself in the company of positive, encouraging people. Limit exposure to toxic relationships and surroundings that drain your energy and resilience. Having a positive network of people around you increases your resilience in the face of hardship.

15. Take Cues from Successful People

Find examples of people who have overcome adversity and study their strategies. Listening to and learning from other people's accounts of overcoming adversity might help you develop your own inner fortitude.

Building Resilience Into Your Routine

Developing resilience is not a one-time effort but a continuing process that involves daily practise and self-awareness. Here are some ideas for increasing resilience that you can use in your daily life:

Morning Reflection: Take a few minutes to think about the day ahead. Determine that you will face difficulties with a can-do attitude and a willingness to learn.

- Mindful Moments: Take frequent, brief pauses to focus on the present moment. Take a few slow, deep breaths to centre yourself.

Reach out to loved ones for comfort and companionship when you feel you need it. The process of establishing a network of allies is never-ending.

Include Self-Care Rituals into your daily life, however you see fit.

 whether that's yoga in the morning, a walk after work, or a weekly trip to the spa. Taking care of yourself in these ways strengthens your mental fortitude.

- Gratitude Practise: On a regular basis, take time to reflect on and celebrate the many blessings in your life. This may enable you to adopt a more optimistic mindset.

- Acts of Kindness: Engage in acts of kindness towards others. Giving to others who are less fortunate can strengthen your own feeling of identity and community, which in turn can strengthen your own resilience.

Final Reflections

The ability to bounce back from adversity and keep one's mental health in check is a hallmark of resilient people. You can cultivate the mindset and abilities to deal with adversity bravely and with hope by adopting simple methods and routines that boost resilience.

Keep in mind that developing resilience is a process that will need time and kindness towards yourself. Having the mental and emotional fortitude to overcome adversity, embrace change, and prosper in spite of life's inherent unpredictability is at the heart of this concept. In the process of taking this journey, you will learn how the trait of resilience may have a profound effect on your mental health for the better.

4.3- Case studies of individuals who have overcome adversity

Exemplary Personal Stories of Perseverance

How people react when faced with adversity often determines who they are and what they become. Throughout history, innumerable individuals have endured immense hurdles, from personal hardships to social barriers, and have not only conquered adversity but also emerged stronger and more resilient. Adaptation is the key to success, and in this we will and over adversity by ad and and and and and adiss sss over adversity, we humans have the power to persevere and even thrive.

Malala Yousafzai: One Girl's Fight for Education in the Face of Persecution

Adversity: When Malala Yousafzai was 15 years old, the Taliban attacked the school bus she was riding in and shot her in the head. The attack was a retaliation to her loud lobbying for girls' education in a province where the Taliban had prohibited it.

Successful Overcoming Malala survived the life-threatening attack, had intensive medical care and rehabilitation, and has since continued her global crusade. In 2014, she was awarded the Nobel Peace Prize, becoming her the youngest person ever to receive this honour. Millions of people around the world are inspired by Malala's persistent commitment to education and gender equality.

Important Takeaways: Malala's courage demonstrates the transformative potential of education and the will to effect positive change in the face of extreme suffering.

Nick Vujicic: Adapting to Life with No Limbs

Adversity: Nick Vujicic was born with tetra-amelia syndrome, which left him without arms or legs. As a child, he faced not only physical obstacles but also social and emotional ones because of his condition.

Successful Overcoming Afraid to let his physical state dictate his life, Nick rejected the idea. He eventually wrote books, gave speeches, and fought for the rights of persons with impairments. Overcoming adversity, bullying, and finding one's own acceptance are topics he has discussed with millions of people around the world. Nick's incredible story of coming to terms with who he is and pushing through difficult times has served as an inspiration to countless people.

Important Takeaways: Nick's story shows how overcoming adversity and developing a strong sense of self-worth and purpose are essential components of true resilience.

From Prisoner to President: Nelson Mandela (3)

Adversity: For 27 years, the apartheid system in South Africa kept Nelson Mandela, an anti-apartheid rebel, in prison. While incarcerated, he was subjected to terrible treatment and was cut off from his loved ones.

Successful Overcoming Nelson Mandela has been an advocate for racial equality and peace ever since he was released from jail in 1990. He was instrumental in the end of apartheid and became the first black president of South Africa in 1994. He led by example, and the nation benefited from his willingness to forgive and make amends.

Important Takeaways: The narrative of Nelson Mandela shows how forgiveness and reconciliation can bring about beneficial cultural transformation in the midst of political persecution.

4. Temple Grandin: Autism Advocate and Innovator

Adversity: Temple Grandin, renowned animal scientist and champion for those with autism, received a diagnosis of the disorder at an early age. She had a hard time talking, feeling comfortable in social situations, and making friends.

Successful Overcoming Temple's autism-inspired perspective and first-hand involvement with the livestock sector ushered in a new era of innovation. Humane animal handling facilities based on her groundbreaking designs are now the norm. Temple has also used her celebrity to promote autism awareness and acceptance. She is now a well-known author and speaker on the topic of neurodiversity.

The main lesson to be learned from Temple Grandin's life is that it is possible to achieve both personal and societal success by embracing one's unique traits and turning adversity into innovation.

J.K. Rowling's Life Story: 5 From Single Parent to Literary Legend

Adversity: J.K. Rowling had to overcome considerable hardships in her own life before she became a household name thanks to her Harry Potter books. She was a young mother raising her child on welfare who was depressed and fighting prejudice towards divorced women.

Successful Overcoming Rowling wrote the first Harry Potter novel because she enjoyed telling stories so much. She persisted even after several publishers turned down her manuscript before one ultimately agreed to publish it. Rowling became one of the most popular authors ever thanks to the unprecedented success of the Harry Potter series.

The moral of J.K. Rowling's story is to follow one's heart no matter the cost and to keep going even when things get tough.

6. Louis Zamperini: Through Unimaginable Adversity

Adversity: During World War II, Olympic athlete and war veteran Louis Zamperini's plane fell into the Pacific Ocean. For 47 days, he and two other survivors were lost at sea and subjected to shark attacks, cold, and hunger until being picked up by the Japanese Navy.

Successful Overcoming Survived the Japanese prisoner-of-war camps and returned to the United States as a Japanese prisoner-of-war. He went on to forgive his captors and became a motivational speaker and author. The life story of a man whose life was the inspiration for the book and film adaptation "Unbroken" centred on the themes of survival, resilience, and forgiveness.

Important Takeaways: Louis Zamperini's life is a powerful example of the transformative power of forgiveness and the resilience of the human spirit in the face of unimaginable adversity.

Number Seven: Oprah Winfrey's Rise from Poverty to Media Power

Adversity: Oprah Winfrey had a difficult childhood filled with trauma and violence as a result of her family's financial struggles. Despite facing racism and sexism on the job, she decided to continue a career in the media.

Successful Overcoming Because of her drive, personality, and work ethic, Oprah has risen to become a global media icon. She was a trailblazer for women and people of colour in Hollywood, and she utilised her fame for good by influencing and motivating millions of others.

Takeaway: Oprah Winfrey's story is an inspiring testament to the power of perseverance, self-belief, and overcoming structural barriers.

Stephen Hawking, 8: Scientific Genius in the Face of Disability

Adversity: Stephen Hawking, one of the world's most known theoretical physicists, was diagnosed with amyotrophic lateral sclerosis (ALS) at the age of 21. He was paralysed and unable to communicate as a result of his illness, and doctors gave him only a few years to live.

Successful Overcoming Hawking maintained his breakthrough research in theoretical physics, contributing significantly to our understanding of the cosmos, despite his physical constraints. He promoted scientific inquiry and astronomy after communicating with a speech-generating gadget.

Important Takeaways: Stephen Hawking's astounding achievements demonstrate the power of persistence, intellect, and dogged pursuit of one's passions despite facing extreme physical difficulty.

Rosa Parks: The Quiet Rebellion That Changed the World

Adversity: In Montgomery, Alabama, Rosa Parks, a seamstress of African descent, encountered racial segregation and prejudice. Her refusal to give up her seat on a segregated bus resulted in her imprisonment on December 1, 1955.

Overcoming Adversity

The Boycott, Divestment, and Sanctions (BDS) movement began as a response to the Rosa Parks' arrest. Her understated defiance sparked a massive and long-lasting movement to end segregation. As a result of the boycott, public buses were desegregated and the civil rights movement advanced.

Important Takeaways: The bravery and perseverance of Rosa Parks show how even modest acts of rebellion may change the world.

10 Christopher Reeve's Superhuman Willpower

Adversity: In 1995, Christopher Reeve, famous for playing Superman in the movies, was paralysed from the neck down after being thrown off his horse.

Successful Overcoming Reeve's paralysis didn't stop him from becoming a champion for spinal cord injury research, though; he established the Christopher Reeve Paralysis Foundation. He was able to restore some feeling and mobility thanks to his own hard work in therapy. His activism helped get more people talking about and giving to research into spinal cord injuries.

Christopher Reeve's unwavering devotion to helping others and his ability to overcome physical difficulties are examples of the strength of the human spirit.

Elizabet Smart, a Fighter for Justice

Adversity: In Salt Lake City, Utah, 14-year-old Elizabeth Smart was kidnapped and imprisoned for nine months. She was abused both physically and psychologically while in captivity.

Successful Overcoming As of the year 2003, Elizabeth Smart had been rescued and was back with her family. She has now dedicated her life to the causes of child protection and post-traumatic growth. To help victims of abduction and sexual exploitation and to bring attention to the problem, she established the Elizabeth Smart Foundation.

Important Takeaways: Resilience, healing, and the capacity to use one's own pain to aid others are all on display in Elizabeth Smart's path from abduction to advocacy.

Winston Churchill, "Leading in Difficult Times"

Adversity: Prime Minister Winston Churchill led the nation through one of the most difficult eras in British history.

In the face of overwhelming odds, the British people were rallied by Churchill's leadership, unwavering resolve, and rousing speeches. He famously stated, "We shall never surrender," and his steadfast commitment helped lead the Allies to victory.

Important Takeaways: Winston Churchill's leadership during World War II is an example of a country's ability to overcome hardship and the transformational potential of visionary leadership.

These examples of people who have overcome misfortune show how the human spirit can overcome extraordinary odds to achieve success. They encourage us to view resiliency as an essential character characteristic that will serve us well in the face of adversity, allow us to develop from our experiences, and make a positive impact on the world.

Despite the fact that each of these people has endured a unique set of challenges, they all have one thing in common: they have refused to let their difficulties define them or bring them down. They serve as a reminder that resilience entails more than just overcoming hardship; it also involves thriving, inspiring others, and leaving a strong and resilient legacy for the generations to come.

Chapter 5:
Practising Kindness to Oneself

5.1- Self-compassion and its role in mental well-being

Importance of Self-Compassion to Overall Health and Happiness

It is more crucial than ever to take care of one's mental health in today's fast-paced and frequently demanding world. The importance of self-compassion in maintaining emotional well-being is often overlooked in the day-to-day grind. Self-compassion is the practise of treating ourselves with the same love and understanding that we would show to a friend facing hardships. It is a potent instrument that plays a crucial part in fostering and maintaining psychological health. We'll break down what self-compassion is, how it can help your mental health, and more.

Learning to Be Kind to Yourself

Mindfulness, the practise of paying attention to one's internal and external sensations without evaluating them, is the foundation of self-compassion. Self-compassion is an interior extension of mindfulness in which one focuses on one's own well-being without judgement or criticism. Dr. Kristin Neff, an early pioneer in the study of self-compassion, has defined the following as the three pillars upon which the concept rests:
1. Self-Kindness: This aspect involves being compassionate and forgiving towards oneself in times of difficulty or while making mistakes. Self-criticism needs to be replaced by self-encouragement and -support. We try to be encouraging and supportive to ourselves rather than critical of our flaws.

2. Common Humanity: In self-compassion, it is crucial to recognise that suffering and difficulties are inherent to the human experience. It's a recognition that we're not the only ones going through tough times. Instead of feeling alone in our suffering, we recognise our common humanity and forge bonds with one another through compassion and understanding.

Mindfulness, the third component, is the practise of paying attention to one's internal experiences without passing judgement on them. This involves accepting our emotions as they are, without trying to change or hide them. Mindfulness helps us develop equanimity in the face of adversity by refocusing our attention on the present moment.

Self-Compassion and Its Importance to Emotional Health

Self-compassion is a potent mental health shield and a growth-inducing force. It has far-reaching consequences, touching on many facets of our psychological well-being:

One benefit of self-compassion is a lessening of the critical thoughts about oneself that can be harmful to mental health. Self-criticism undermines our confidence and happiness, but self-kindness does quite the opposite.
Researchers have found that self-compassion has a negative correlation with depressive and anxious states. Mood problems are less common in people who regularly practise self-compassion.

Thirdly, self-compassion increases one's ability to bounce back quickly from setbacks. It encourages resilience by teaching people to see challenges with curiosity and a willingness to improve.

Improved emotional regulation is a fourth benefit of practising self-compassion. Emotional distress can be mitigated by the practise of mindfulness and self-kindness, which encourages us to accept and acknowledge our feelings.

5. Greater Happiness and Satisfaction with Life: Research suggests that practising self-compassion might lead to more contentment and joy in one's daily life. Individuals tend to enjoy more well-being when they are treated with compassion and acceptance.

In a surprising twist, self-compassion can actually serve as a driving force for personal development. Recognising our flaws without condemnation paves the way for self-improvement.

Self-compassion has been shown to have beneficial effects on interpersonal interactions. The ability to accept and care for oneself increases, as does the likelihood of developing meaningful relationships with one's peers.

Methods That Actually Work To Improve Your Self-Compassion
Self-compassion is a talent that may be honed with practise; nevertheless, it is a slow and continual process. Here are some concrete steps you may take to cultivate self-compassion and enjoy its positive effects on your mental health:

1. Mindful Self-Compassion Meditation: Engage in mindfulness meditation activities specifically designed to foster self-compassion. These guided meditations can help you become more compassionate and accepting of yourself.

2. Write a Self-Compassion Letter: Picture yourself penning a letter to a close friend who is going through something similar to what you're going through. Be encouraging and sympathetic in your words. Then, have a private reading of the letter.

Third, Pay Attention To And Challenge Your Inner Critic. Consider if your words would be acceptable if you were speaking to a close friend. Substitute self-compassion with self-criticism.

Recognise that everyone is fallible and has difficulties; this is what we mean by "Common Humanity." Remember that you are not alone in having problems when you make a mistake. Recognise that you, like everyone else, are flawed.

5. Use Self-Compassion Mantras: Create meaningful mantras or affirmations to help you practise self-compassion. In the face of adversity or doubt, remind yourself of these positive statements.
6. Engage in Self-Care: Prioritise self-care activities that nourish your mind, body, and soul. Some examples are working out, sitting quietly, writing in a journal, or going for a walk in the park.

Sharing your struggles and feelings with a trusted friend, family member, or mental health professional can help you manage difficult emotions and get support. Self-compassion can be strengthened by receiving the support and sympathy of others.

Regardless of how insignificant you may think your successes are, it is important to recognise and honour them. Recognising your progress improves confidence and self-compassion.

Set goals that are within your reach, and if necessary, be willing to change them. Don't put unnecessary pressure on yourself by holding to unrealistic expectations.

Forget about previous mistakes and regrets by practising self-forgiveness. Keep in mind that you are human, and that your mistakes are not indicative of your value.

Instances of Self-Compassion in Real Life

Let's look at some real-life people who have embraced self-compassion and benefited from it:

1. Tara Brach, Author and Mindfulness Instructor

Tara Brach is an accomplished author and meditation instructor who has guided many people towards greater self-acceptance through the cultivation of mindfulness. In this regard, she stresses the value of self-awareness and the cultivation of self-compassion. Her lectures and writings, such as "Radical Acceptance," have helped many people learn to be kinder to themselves and improve their quality of life.

2. Dr. Bre

Susan Brown: Expert on Vulnerability and Guilt

Dr. Brené Brown is an academic whose writings and studies have focused extensively on the topics of exposure, shame, and recovery. Her study shows that self-compassion is key to letting go of shame and building self-esteem. Her books and TED talks have encouraged many people to take risks and be kind to themselves as ways to improve their mental health.

Dr. Kristin Neff, a forerunner in the field of self-compassion research

As was previously noted, Dr. Kristin Neff is a trailblazer in the study of self-compassion. The concept of self-compassion and its advantages for mental health have been clarified because to her considerable research. She provides tools to help people build self-compassion and has created exercises and evaluations to gauge self-compassion.
Self-compassion is gaining popularity in the celebrity world.
Many well-known people have spoken candidly about the necessity of self-compassion in dealing with mental health issues. Both Demi Lovato and Prince Harry have utilised their platforms to encourage self-compassion and lessen the stigma associated with mental well-being, with Lovato focusing on self-love and acceptance and the prince focusing on raising awareness about mental health.

Conclusion

When practised regularly, self-compassion can be a potent antidote to negative thought patterns including harsh self-criticism, perfectionism, and judgement. Self-compassion entails being as patient and forgiving with oneself as one would be with a friend who was going through a tough time. Reducing anxiety and despair, boosting resilience, and encouraging improved well-being are all possible through practising self-compassion.

Self-compassion is not something you achieve once and then forget about. To do so, we must be present, aware, and dedicated to treating ourselves kindly and compassionately, even in the face of adversity. By making self-compassion a regular practise, we may harness the transformative power of this deceptively basic idea and lay the groundwork for enduring mental health. Self-compassion is a priceless present you can offer yourself, therefore always keep in mind that you deserve kindness.

5.2- Practical exercises for self-compassion

Self-Compassion: Practicable Methods

Practising self-compassion is a potent and life-altering activity that can greatly improve one's emotional health. It entails being as sympathetic to your own plight as you would be to that of a close friend who is experiencing difficulties. It may not come naturally, but self-compassion is a skill that can be honed and improved with practise. Fortunately, self-compassion may be fostered via the regular practise of specific exercises and strategies. Several methods for cultivating and refining self-compassion are discussed below.

1 A Letter of Compassion for Oneself

Self-compassion can be fostered through the practise of writing a self-compassion letter. Take the time to compose a letter to yourself as you would to a close friend who is struggling. Share your sympathy and words of support. Recognise your difficulties and comfort yourself that you are human and hence allowed to make mistakes. When you need a dose of self-compassion, reading this letter can be very soothing.

Mantras and affirmations for self-compassion are up next.

Make a collection of words of wisdom or affirmations that you can repeat to yourself as a form of self-compassion. These are short, encouraging words that you can repeat to yourself in moments of self-doubt or self-criticism. Use of the word paraphrase in a sentence.

- "I am worthy of love and compassion, just as I am."
- "I embrace my imperfections with kindness and understanding."
- "I am allowed to make mistakes; they do not define my worth."
- "I treat myself with the same compassion I would offer to a friend."

Get in the habit of using affirmations every day by picking ones that really speak to you. Use them every morning and night, or whenever you feel you need an extra dose of compassion for yourself.

3. Mindful Self-Compassion Meditation 3. Mindful Self-Compassion Meditation

Self-compassion can be developed and strengthened through the practise of mindfulness meditation. Practise a guided meditation on being kind to yourself mindfully. In this meditation, you'll give yourself permission to feel whatever you're feeling and think whatever you're thinking without passing judgement. It's a method for training oneself to have more compassionate thoughts and feelings.

4. A Sense of Our Shared Humanity

Learn to see the humanity in others and accept it. Keep in mind that you are not alone in encountering obstacles or failing at something. Think on the idea that you're not the only one going through this. Understanding this can help you feel less alone by increasing your capacity for empathy and compassion.

Take on your inner critic. 5.

how to recognise the critical voice inside your head and how to quiet it. When you catch yourself thinking negatively, ask yourself:

- "Would I say these things to a friend?"
- "Is this criticism based on facts, or is it distorted by negative self-perception?"
- "What would be a more compassionate and balanced way to view this situation?"

One way to change one's perspective and lessen self-critical tendencies is to challenge one's inner critic.

6. The Self-Compassion Break

Practising this technique can be especially helpful while facing difficulties. Take a self-compassion break whenever you're in a trying or stressful situation:

First, practise mindfulness by being aware of the pain you're in and the difficulty of the present moment. Remind yourself, "This is a moment of suffering."

Second, Common Humanity: Keep in mind that pain is inherent to being human. As an explanation, you could remark, "Life is full of suffering. In this, I know I am not alone.

Third, practise self-kindness by speaking kindly and compassionately to oneself. Use phrases such, "May I treat myself kindly. I pray that I will be able to show myself some kindness.

This straightforward practise can ease your suffering in an instant and teach you to be more compassionate to yourself when facing difficulties.

Journaling for self-compassion (7)

Keep a self-compassion journal to record your thoughts and feelings as you work towards greater self-compassion. Write down in your notebook the times you were very compassionate and nice to yourself, as well as the times you were hard on yourself. The journal can be used for introspection, the establishment of self-compassion objectives, and the subsequent celebration of one's progress towards those objectives.

Seek Support and Connection. 8. Seek Support and Connection.

If you feel like you need someone to talk to or someone who can help you comprehend what you're going through, don't be afraid to do so. Having someone to talk to about your problems and emotions might help you feel less alone and increase your capacity for compassion and empathy.

9. Practise Self-Care

Maintain your mental and physical health by partaking in self-care practises on a regular basis. Physical exercise and meditation are just two examples; others include reading, hiking, and pursuing other interests. When you put yourself first and do things that make you feel good, you are practising self-compassion.

Mindful breathing and self-compassion are 10 on the list.

When practised in conjunction with self-compassion, mindful breathing proves to be a powerful tool. If you're feeling overwhelmed, try meditating for a few minutes. Repeat affirmations or words of self-compassion as you take deep breaths in and out, such as:

- "I breathe in peace and exhale self-criticism."
- "With each breath, I cultivate self-kindness and understanding."
- "In this moment, I am worthy of compassion and love."

The Eleventh Step: Forgive Yourself

Forgive yourself for whatever wrongdoings or regrets you may have. Recognise that blunders are inevitable and in no way indicative of your value. Allow yourself to go forward with self-compassion by letting go of guilt and self-blame.

12 Establish Practical Objectives and Predictions

Try to keep your expectations in check and focus on achieving the goals you set. Avoid setting too high standards that can lead to self-criticism and disillusionment. Accept that failures and lessons are necessary components of growth and development.

Celebrate the Little Victories

No matter how insignificant they may seem, acknowledge and rejoice in your successes. Taking the time to acknowledge and appreciate even the smallest of accomplishments may do wonders for your self-esteem. It's a great method to cultivate kindness towards oneself.

The Relationship Between Mindful Eating and Self-Compassion

Mindful eating mixed with self-compassion can help you overcome negative thoughts about food and your body. Do not pass judgement on your body as you learn to listen to its signals of hunger and fullness. Be gentle and forgiving with yourself; your value is not based on how you look or what you eat.

Prepare a self-compassion ritual for 15 on the list.

Develop a self-care practise that you can do regularly, whether it's once a week or every day. It might be as easy as lighting a candle, repeating kind words to yourself, or sitting quietly for a while. Creating a routine helps you stay committed to self-care.

Use Visualisation Methods. 16.

Think of someone or something who brings you comfort and compassion, whether it be a real person, a spiritual guide, or a fictional character. The figure appears to you and offers words of kindness, understanding, and support. As you can see, this diagram facilitate the emergence of self-compassion in times of need.

Take a workshop or class on self-compassion. 17.

Think about enrolling in a self-compassion course taught by professionals or therapists. These seminars provide opportunity to develop your understanding of self-compassion and engage in guided exercises with people who share similar goals.

18 Record Audio Messages of Self-Compassion

Create an audio file in which you speak kind and encouraging words to yourself. Listen to these affirmations when you're having a hard time believing in yourself or accepting help from others.

Keep in mind that nurturing self-compassion is a process that will take time and care towards yourself. It's normal to experience some resistance or self-criticism while you work through these exercises, so be easy on yourself. Self-compassion has a huge effect on one's mental health, and it can be fostered with effort and time. With practise, self-compassion can become second nature, allowing you to face adversity with more strength and gentleness towards yourself.

5.3- The connection between self-compassion and resilience

Self-Compassion and Perseverance: A Powerful Combo

The capacity to persevere in the face of adversity, or resilience, is highly valued in today's society. The ability to persevere, adapt, and evolve in the face of adversity is frequently the defining factor in one's sense of well-being in the face of life's many challenges, setbacks, and unexpected turns. Self-compassion is a potent and underappreciated aspect in promoting resilience.

Resilience is intricately connected with self-compassion, the practise of treating oneself with care and understanding. It provides the emotional and psychological support necessary to weather life's storms and emerge stronger. The ability to deal with misfortune depends in large part on our capacity for self-compassion, and we'll discuss how self-compassion training can help you develop that capacity.

What You Need to Know About Resilience

Our ability to bounce back from setbacks, stress, and major life problems is part of what makes us resilient; it is not a static trait. It consists of the following central components:

Resilience shines brightest in the face of adversity, which can take many forms, such as difficulties one must overcome on an individual basis, trauma, loss, or major life changes.

To be resilient, one must be able to get themselves up after being knocked down by hardship. Resilience is not the absence of emotional upheaval, but rather the ability to recover from negative states of mind.

Third, the ability to change and develop as a result of adversity is an essential part of resilience; without it, recuperation alone would not be enough. It can be a springboard to better judgement, more resilience, and overall development.

4. Support Systems: Whether it comes from friends and family, a sense of community, or your own inner strength, a robust support system is an essential part of being resilient. These support systems provide the necessary emotional resources to weather adversities.

5. Coping Strategies: People who are able to bounce back from adversity successfully use a variety of coping mechanisms, including creative problem-solving, reaching out for support, and making the best of a bad situation.

The Building Blocks of Self-Compassion

Dr. Kristin Neff's definition of self-compassion includes three interconnected factors:

First, Self-Kindness: When you practise self-compassion, you show yourself the same compassion you'd show a good friend. It entails showing compassion and support for oneself in the face of adversity rather than condemnation.

A major feature of self-compassion is the recognition that suffering and challenges are part of the human experience. To do this, we must accept that our challenges are shared by others and that human imperfection is a fact of life.

Third, we have something called "mindfulness," which involves looking at one's inner world without passing judgement. It entails keeping an objective distance from one's own thoughts and feelings rather than trying to suppress or suppress them.

Self-compassion and resiliency: a dynamic duo

Self-compassion is an important trigger for resilience, and the relationship between the two is intricate and nuanced. Here's where these ideas meet and how they strengthen one another:

1) Emotional Control and Adaptation

Emotional control is improved through self-compassion because it offers a more constructive method to deal with emotional stress and anguish. Self-compassion is the ability to recognise and accept one's own emotional suffering while also responding to it with warmth and acceptance. This kind of empathetic reaction to pain eases mental anguish and makes it easier for people to deal with adversity.

Second, "Lessening One's Own Criticism"

Self-criticism is a major roadblock to resilience. Harsh self-judgment and self-blame can increase the impact of hardship and delay healing. Self-compassion is a proactive response to self-criticism that helps people learn to treat themselves with kindness rather than judgement. This new outlook encourages self-love and forgiving, which in turn increases resilience.

Improving Confidence in One's Capabilities

Self-compassion boosts self-efficacy, or confidence in one's own abilities to handle adversity. When people face challenges with kindness and understanding for themselves, they strengthen their belief in their own resilience. They have a fundamental belief in their inherent value that allows them to persevere and change in the face of hardship.

4. Promoting Positive Growth

To be resilient is to grow and change as a person rather than simply bounce back to health after hardship. Post-adversity growth is facilitated by self-compassion, which enables people to find significance and lessons in their circumstances. Individuals can grow from misfortune by compassionately accepting themselves, flaws and all, and learning to use them to their advantage.

5. Establishing Mutually Beneficial Connections

Building strong bonds with others and a solid support system is an integral part of practising self-compassion. When people are compassionate and patient with themselves, they are less likely to feel ashamed about asking for help. Their social networks, an integral part of resilience, are bolstered as a result.

6. Reducing Psychological Distress

Lower Anxiety and Depression: Are They Linked? Lower Anxiety and Depression: Are They Linked? The emotional toll of adversity can be lessened by cultivating a self-compassionate perspective, which in turn facilitates recovery and adaptation.

Methods to Foster Self-Compassion and Perseverance

The ability to practise self-compassion can be honed with regular effort. Methods to foster self-compassion and increase resilience include the following:

Meditation with Kindness to Oneself (Mindful Self-Compassion)

Participate in guided meditations that promote conscious self-compassion. These methods encourage a warm and accepting examination of one's inner experience. Self-compassion is a skill worth cultivating, and guided meditations with that intention might be helpful.

2. Self-Compassion Journaling

Keep a self-compassion journal to document your progress in developing compassion for yourself. Think of times when you were patient and understanding with yourself while you worked through difficult situations. Keeping a journal is a great way to monitor your development and spot potential problem areas.

Letters of self-compassion

Compose letters of kindness and understanding to yourself in the same way you would to a close friend. Send comforting words of sympathy, support, and reassurance. These letters are a physical manifestation of your ability to practise self-compassion.

Mindful breathing and self-compassion (4)

Take a few deep breaths and tell yourself kind things whenever you feel overwhelmed. While breathing in and out, you could tell yourself something like, "I breathe in self-compassion; I exhale self-criticism."

5. Confront Your Inner Critic

Learn to identify your inner critic and actively counter negative beliefs. Consider if your words would be acceptable if you were speaking to a close friend. Substitute self-compassion and understanding for self-criticism.

6 Mandalas and Affirmations for Self-Compassion

Create personal mantras or affirmations to help you practise self-compassion. Use these positive statements as mantras to recite upon waking, before going to sleep, or whenever you're feeling down. Make changes to suit your own self-compassion objectives.

7. Mindful Eating and Self-Compassion

If you have concerns with how you seem in the mirror or with your eating habits,

mix self-compassion with mindful eating. Recognise that your value is independent of your appearance and eating habits, and pay heed to your body's signals without passing judgement on them.

8. Look for Friends and Allies

When you're feeling down, don't be shy about reaching out for help from loved ones or a professional in the field of mental health. Talking to other people about your struggles is a great way to build resilience and strengthen your practise of self-compassion.

9 Celebrate Mini-Successes

No matter how insignificant they may seem, acknowledge and rejoice in your successes. Taking stock of your accomplishments and celebrating them can do wonders for your self-esteem. It's a great method to cultivate kindness towards oneself.

10. Rituals of Self-Compassion

Create self-care rituals that you can perform once a week or once a day. Simple acts like lighting a candle, repeating kind words to oneself, or sitting quietly to reflect are all examples of meaningful rituals.

Real-Life Illustrations of Resilience and Self-Compassion

The strong relationship between self-compassion and resilience is demonstrated by several real-world examples:

Advocate for Girls' Education 1. Malala Yousafzai

Pakistani feminist Malala Yousafzai was shot by the Taliban for speaking out in favour of girls' education. Malala shown incredible perseverance in the face of adversity. She overcame adversity to become a global advocate for girls' rights because she had compassion for herself, as evidenced by her unyielding belief in her cause and dedication to education.

2. Nelson Mandela: Leader of Peace and Reconciliation

For his part in the anti-apartheid movement in South Africa, Nelson Mandela was imprisoned for 27 years. The power of self-compassion is demonstrated by his ability to forgive and reconcile after serving time in prison. With his ability to forgive himself and others, Mandela paved the way for a peaceful end to apartheid in South Africa.

3. Maya Angelou, Indomitable Poet and Writer

Maya Angelou, acclaimed poet and author, suffered great difficulties in her life, including childhood trauma and racial persecution. She credited her ability to persevere to her capacity for self-compassion. Through introspection, self-compassion, and expressive writing, Angelou was able to discover meaning and healing in her life's events.

Holocaust survivor and psychologist Dr. Victor Frankl is our 4 Through his ability to find meaning in his suffering, Holocaust survivor and famous psychologist Victor Frankl shown remarkable endurance. His time spent in a concentration camp inspired him to create logotherapy, a method of therapy that centres on the pursuit of meaning. In the midst of inconceivable adversity, Frankl's capacity to nurture self-compassion and find inner strength was the foundation of his resilience.

Conclusion

The ability to bounce back from setbacks and even thrive in challenging situations is a key component of resilience. The ability to treat oneself with empathy and compassion, known as self-compassion, is crucial in fostering resilience. Developing a compassionate attitude towards oneself helps us face life's difficulties with more strength and perseverance.

Self-compassion and resilience are inextricably linked, with the former supporting the latter. Self-compassion is an essential part of building resilience because it lessens negative self-talk, helps you keep your emotions in check, boosts your confidence, and encourages you to develop as a person. We may strengthen our resilience and meet hardship with more strength, wisdom, and grace by actively practising self-compassion through mindfulness, self-kindness, and acceptance.

Keep in mind that self-compassion and resilience are abilities that can be honed and improved with time and practise as you set out on your path. Have compassion for oneself and acknowledge the universal experiences of fallibility and development. The ability to persevere through adversity and emerge stronger and more whole is a direct result of cultivating self-compassion.

Chapter 6:
Mindful Interaction and Communication

6.1- Mindful communication in personal and professional relationships

Relational and Professional Benefits of Mindful Communication

Relationships, whether personal or professional, can't function without effective communication. Poor communication can lead to misunderstandings, conflict, and strained relationships, while good communication can promote understanding, connection, and collaboration. Mindful communication has been widely recognised as an effective method for enhancing the quality of interpersonal interactions and relationships in recent years.

Being fully present in talks, listening carefully, and responding with awareness and purpose are all aspects of mindful communication. It's based on the mindfulness tenets of acceptance, openness, and kindness in the present moment. This article will introduce the concept of mindful communication, its guiding principles, and some methods for putting them into practise in both personal and professional contexts.

The Value of Reflective Speech
Communicating effectively is about more than simply getting your point through; it's also about building relationships and getting to know the other person. Mindful communication may have a significant effect in every environment, from personal interactions with loved ones to professional interactions with coworkers and clients.

One benefit of communicating mindfully is increased comprehension since it promotes attentive listening. Being present in the moment increases one's odds of picking up on subtleties in a conversation.

Conflicts can be avoided and resolved via considerate conversation. Individuals can discover common ground and work towards solutions that benefit all parties if they approach arguments with understanding and sensitivity.

3. Improved Relationships: Mindful communication strengthens relationships by establishing an atmosphere of trust, respect, and open discourse. Connection and empathy on an emotional level are fostered, both of which are necessary for happy partnerships.

Increased empathy results from practising mindful communication, which opens one up to the ideas and emotions of others. Having this kind of compassion and connection with others is fostered by empathy.

Leadership that gets results: 5. Mindful communication is an essential leadership quality in the business world. Leaders who pay attention to their words have a better chance of gaining their employees' respect and following them with clarity and compassion. The sixth benefit of mindful communication is a decrease in stress, which is beneficial in both personal and professional settings. By approaching talks with mindfulness and calm, individuals can lessen the emotional toll of tough exchanges.

Important Guidelines for Mindful Interaction

Paradoxically, the values of compassion are firmly based in the ideas of present. Important guidelines for communicating with awareness:

1. Present-Moment Awareness: Mindful Communication calls for one to provide one's undivided attention to the activity at hand. In other

words, you should stop what you're doing and pay attention to the person you're talking to instead than trying to juggle many tasks at once.

Non-Judgmental Presence: Enter Conversations Without Judgement 2. Don't jump to conclusions about the other person's motivations or attitude based on what they say or do.

3. Deep Listening: Make it a habit to listen carefully, taking into account not just the words being spoken, but also the speaker's tone, body language, and emotional state. Listen carefully without forming questions or comments in your thoughts.

Empathetic Reaction 4: Be understanding and sympathetic in your reply. Listen to the other person and validate their thoughts and experiences. Reflect their feelings and thoughts to demonstrate comprehension and empathy.

5. Mindful Speech: Watch your own words carefully. Choose your words carefully, talk honestly and gently, and consider the impact of your words on the other person. Talk and act in a way that won't injure others.

6 Pause and Reflect: Think about how you want to respond before immediately answering a remark or inquiry. Taking that time will help you reply thoughtfully, rather than reflexively. Conflicts and misunderstandings can be avoided as a result.

Cultivate empathy and compassion in your interactions with others. 7. Realise that the other person is a feeling, thinking, willing, and needing human being, just like you are. Sincere desire for actual understanding of how to relate with others.

Practical Strategies for Mindful Communication

Now that we've covered the foundational concepts behind mindful communication, let's dive into some concrete methods for putting them to use in our everyday lives.

1. Mindful Listening: Pay close attention to what the other person is saying. Try not to think of what you're going to say in response while the other person is still talking. Focus on understanding their perspective.

2. Mindful Presence: Give your whole attention to the people you're talking to. Put away any electronic gadgets you may be using and focus on the other person. This demonstrates that you recognise the importance of their feedback.

Thirdly, Non-Verbal Expression: Consider the significance of body language and facial expressions in addition to words. These signs typically reveal feelings and intentions that may not be expressed explicitly. Paying attention to non-verbal cues helps you grasp what's being said.

To guarantee you have understood the other person's words, use reflective listening by restating them in your own words. For example, you can say, "So, if I understand you correctly, you're saying that..."

5. Compassionate Reactions: Be understanding and sympathetic in your reply. You can show that you care about the other person and their feelings by saying something like, "I can see why you might feel that way" or "I understand why you're upset." Demonstrate empathy for how they're feeling.

Mindful Speech (6): Watch what you say. Be careful what you say, especially in tense or argumentative situations. Instead of using accusatory or blaming language, try expressing your thoughts, feelings, and needs in "I" statements.

Pause before reacting to a challenging or emotionally charged situation. 7. Pause before reacting to a challenging or emotionally charged situation. This pause will give you time to gather your thoughts, suppress any knee-jerk reactions, and respond thoughtfully.

8. Express Gratitude: Do this in your personal and professional interactions. Recognising the efforts and talents of others creates a more upbeat and receptive environment.

If you don't understand what the other person has said, ask them to elaborate by using open-ended inquiries. Don't presume anything or rush to judgement.

10 Always Be Receptive to Feedback: Listen to the comments and suggestions of those around you. Instead than seeing criticism, view it as input for future development.

Relationships are strengthened when feedback is accepted thoughtfully.

When disagreements happen, try approaching them with attentive dialogue and a calm demeanour. Instead of assigning blame, try to get at the true nature of the problems and feelings at play. Find answers that work for both of you.

The importance of having well-defined limits in both personal and professional relationships cannot be overstated. You should be assertive and calm while communicating your boundaries, and you should respect the boundaries of others.
Extend the benefits of mindful communication to yourself by engaging in self-compassion. 13. Treat yourself with the same love and understanding you provide to others, especially in moments of self-criticism or doubt.

In business contexts, it's important to hold meetings with a focus on being present and thoughtful. Establish ground rules for involvement and active listening. See to ensuring that everyone gets a chance to share their thoughts.

15. Feedback and Recognition: Be thoughtful while giving and receiving feedback and acknowledgment in professional settings. Recognise and applaud your coworkers' successes, and be constructive in your criticism.

Learn and practise conflict resolution strategies that are in line with the concepts of mindful communication, such as active listening, I-statements, and the pursuit of win-win solutions.

Mindful Communication: Real-Life Examples

In both personal and professional settings, real-world examples show how attentive communication can make a world of a difference.

Couples Therapy: 1. In a problematic marriage, a couple sought counselling to enhance their connection. They were able to better comprehend one other's points of view and begin to reestablish trust by practising mindful communication strategies like active listening and empathic answers.

 2. Team Collaboration: In a business setting, a cross-functional team experienced difficulties in communicating, which resulted in conflicts and delays. Improved teamwork and output were the results of a shift towards more mindful communication practises including mindful meetings and active listening.

One parent who had trouble communicating with their adolescent child tried instead to focus on the present moment when talking to their child. The parent established a more honest and trusting relationship with their child by listening attentively, offering sympathy, and without passing judgement.

4. Workplace Conflict Resolution: Mindful conversation was the key to solving a problem between coworkers. A compromise was reached and the parties' working relationship was strengthened as a result of their reciprocal efforts to listen thoughtfully and get each other's perspective.

Conclusion

Communicating mindfully is a life-changing skill that can improve all of your interactions, both personal and professional. Understanding, trust, and empathy can flourish when people connect with one another in accordance with the tenets of mindfulness, which include paying attention in the here and now, suspending judgement, and showing kindness.

Mindful communication isn't only good for the moment; it also helps build stronger bonds between people over time. By practising mindful communication, we can build understanding, settle disagreements, and enhance our ties with others. Intimately and professionally Paraphrase is a strong tool for managing the complexity of interpersonal interactions.

6.2- Navigating conflict with mindfulness

Conflict Resolution Through Mindfulness

Conflict arises in all human interactions, whether amongst friends, in the workplace, or between neighbours. Conflict is not inherently bad, but how we respond to it and handle it can have a major impact on our happiness and the quality of our relationships. When used to conflict resolution, mindfulness's emphasis on acceptance and acceptance of one's experience provides a useful foundation. The principles of mindful conflict resolution, as well as concrete techniques for incorporating mindfulness into conflict resolution, and concrete experiences demonstrating its transforming power, will be discussed in this article.

Conflict Resolution

Disagreement happens when two or more parties have opposing goals, values, or worldviews. Disagreement comes in all shapes and sizes, from the superficial to the systemic. Examples of typical causes of tension are:

Misunderstandings can misinterpretations which can in turn misinterpretations which can mislead.

- Competing Interests: When individuals or groups have conflicting goals or interests, it can result in friction.

Personal insecurities, painful memories, and other emotional triggers can all lead to heightened levels of conflict.

Values and beliefs that are at odds with one another can lead to ideological or cultural friction.

Conflicts can be fueled by the struggle for scarce resources like time, money, and opportunity.

The Role of Mindfulness in Conflict Resolution

By encouraging introspection, emotional stability, and sympathetic exchanges, mindfulness offers a potent theoretical foundation for dealing with contentious situations. It encourages people to think about the following guidelines whenever they engage in conflict:

Present-Moment Awareness: Mindfulness teaches people to be in the here-and-now, noticing their thoughts, feelings, and bodily sensations without judgement when they experience a conflict. This understanding allows people to respond intentionally rather than reflexively.

2. Non-Judgmental Presence: Mindfulness encourages people to resist from labelling or blaming themselves or others during times of conflict. An accepting demeanour encourages receptivity and empathy.

3. Empathetic Understanding: Mindfulness fosters empathy by training one to put oneself in the shoes of another and experience what it's like to feel what they feel. This insight inspires caring reactions and a desire to work together.

4. Emotional Regulation: Mindfulness practises aid in controlling one's emotional reactions to tense situations. Individuals can respond to conflict with more emotional balance if they learn to recognise and accept their feelings without becoming attached to them.

5. Non-Reactivity: Mindfulness teaches people to take a moment to calm down and think things through before reacting to a challenging situation. They can take a breather and decide how to respond rationally rather than emotionally.

Effective Methods for Dealing with Conflict Mindfully

Using mindfulness to resolve conflicts calls for an integration of introspection, compassion, and open dialogue. The following are some helpful guidelines for avoiding and resolving conflicts:

Self-awareness () Get to know yourself first. Learn to identify your own personal conflict-related emotional triggers, prejudices, and habitual reactions. Recognise that your reactions may be influenced by your past experiences.

Second, practise mindful breathing to keep yourself centred and composed in tense situations. Learn to control your feelings and make room for measured answers by focusing on your breathing.

3. Active Listening: Give the other person your undivided attention while you listen to them. Don't try to think of an answer or interrupt them while they're talking. Consider their point of view instead.

Keep a non-defensive posture (both physically and psychologically) at all times. Keep your arms at your sides, look people in the eye, and listen to what they have to say.

Use introspective comments to validate the other person's thoughts and perspective when it is your chance to speak. 5. Attempt a phrase like, "I can understand why you feel that way."

6 Pause and Reflect: Think about how you want to respond before immediately answering a remark or inquiry. Don't forget the weight of your words. This delay helps curb hasty responses.

7. I-Statements: Instead of saying "you" or "they," say "I" or "my" to convey your emotions and requirements. Instead of saying "You always..." try "I feel frustrated when..."

Empathetic Questions 8. Ask compassionate questions to obtain a deeper knowledge of the other person's perspective. Let's say "Can you help me understand why this is important to you?"

Past and Future Conflicts: Avoiding the Future by Living in the Past and the Future by Avoiding the Present. Don't lose track of the here-and-now discussion or the topics at hand.

10. Set Boundaries: Clearly explain your boundaries and expectations in the dispute resolution process. Honour the personal space of those around you.

Consider involving a neutral mediator or facilitator to lead the process and ensure a fair conclusion in circumstances of serious or prolonged dispute (see 11, "Seek Mediation").

12. Conflict as Growth Opportunity: Think of fights as chances to learn and grow as a person and in your relationships. Think of it as an opportunity to learn and explore new things.

Take some time for mindful closure after settling a disagreement. Think about how you can use your newfound knowledge in future conversations.

Practical Conflict Resolution Strategies

Examples from real life show how mindful conflict resolution may turn problems into learning experiences:

1. Family Conflict Resolution: Members of a family dealing with generational tensions and strained communications engaged in regular sessions of mindful conflict resolution. They patched things up by giving each other their full attention and treating their differences with compassion.

2. Workplace Mediation: In a business context, a group's internal issues were getting in the way of their ability to work together effectively. Team members learnt to communicate more effectively through the use of mindful conflict resolution led by a trained mediator, which enhanced teamwork and outcomes.

3. Marital Harmony: A married couple with persistent disagreements sought out couples counselling that emphasised the use of mindfulness techniques. By learning to pause and ponder before reacting, communicate their feelings honestly, and empathetically listen to one other, they restored harmony in their marriage.

4. Community Dialogue: In a community coping with cultural conflicts and divisive problems, community leaders organised mindfulness-based talks. Participants were able to have frank, judgment-free interactions in these settings, leading to increased mutual understanding and cooperation.

Conclusion

Conflict is inevitable in interpersonal interactions, but how we respond to it has far-reaching consequences. By putting an emphasis on self-awareness, empathy, and intentional communication, mindful approaches to conflict resolution can have a profound impact. By adopting the concepts of mindfulness—present-moment awareness, non-judgmental presence, sympathetic understanding, emotion control, and non-reactivity—we may negotiate conflict in a more productive and compassionate manner.

Methods in the real world for

Listening attentively, thinking before speaking, remaining neutral, and establishing limits are all part of resolving conflicts mindfully. Using these methods, people can turn negative interactions into learning experiences that strengthen relationships and personal development.

Mindful conflict resolution has been shown to be effective in a variety of settings, from the home and interpersonal interactions to the business and the larger community. Using mindfulness to resolve conflicts helps us stop reacting emotionally and instead respond rationally, empathically, and compassionately. Ultimately, being conscious when resolving conflicts helps bring about more peace, better connections, and development on all fronts.

6.3- Building supportive networks

Strengthening Existing Connections

Humans have an innate need to interact with others. When we interact with people, learn from one another, and form bonds, we flourish. Having a strong social network is important for our health and success in both our personal and professional lives. In this article, we will discuss the importance of developing supportive networks, tactics for cultivating and maintaining these networks, and the benefits they give in numerous facets of our life.

The Value of Caring Relationships

Social support systems, or supportive networks, consist of the people in our lives who care about us and who we care about. There are many ways in which these connections are essential to our existence:

1. Emotional Well-Being: Having a strong social network can help you cope with difficult emotions like stress, loss, or boredom when facing difficult situations in life. Knowing that there are others rooting for us might lighten the load we carry emotionally.

Improved mental health is one of the many benefits of having strong social ties. Anxiety, sadness, and other mental health difficulties can be better managed with the help of a strong support system that listens and cares.

Opportunity for development and enhancement in oneself can be found in a network of people who care about you. When we surround ourselves with supportive people like friends, mentors, and coworkers, we increase our chances of reaching our full potential.

Professional Success 4. Having a group of people who have your back at work may do wonders for your professional growth, happiness at work, and chances of getting promoted. Building relationships with contemporaries and role models can lead to novel opportunities and fruitful partnerships.

Stress and feelings of being overwhelmed are lessened when one realises they have people they can rely on for assistance. Supportive networks give a safety net during hard times.

Physical Studies have demonstrated that a favourable influence on mental health has a positive impact on physical health. Better immune function and lower risk of chronic diseases have both been linked to the presence of strong social support systems.

Resilience, or the capacity to overcome hardship, is bolstered by the presence of a strong social network. Strength in adversity comes from surrounding yourself with people who support you and believe in you.

Strategies for Cultivating Supportive Networks

A dynamic process, network development and maintenance requires conscious effort and the nurturing of relationships. Here are some methods for developing and solidifying such connections:

Determine Your Specific Requirements: Think about what you need help with specifically. Think about whether you need someone to talk to, someone to guide you in your work, a mentor, or all three. If you know what you need, you can focus on the correct people.

Make Contact with People You Already Know: Start by using your existing connections. Get in touch with people you know you can trust, such as close relatives, friends, and coworkers. Tell them about your plans, obstacles, and hopes.

3. Networking: Make the most of professional and personal opportunities to meet new people and expand your professional network. Go to functions, conferences, and social gatherings to make connections and meet new people.

Join groups and communities that share your interests and aspirations, whether they be in person or virtual. A common bond can be established through shared interests.

5. Be Sincere and Real: True honesty is essential to developing trusting friendships. Act naturally and with sincere curiosity in others. The are more ever and ever ever ever ever and ever.

6. Provide Assistance: Creating helpful connections is a two-way street. Don't be hesitant to lend a helping hand to those who need it. Relationships are strengthened by acts of generosity and reciprocity.

7 Look for Mentors: Locate people who may serve as role models for your career and/or personal growth. Mentors offer insightful advise, positive reinforcement, and perspective.

Communicate effectively by working on your abilities regularly. Pay close attention, inquire thoughtfully, and show sympathy when someone else is talking about a difficulty or an event they've had.

9. Grow Preexisting Connections: Don't ignore the people who are already in your life. Keep in touch with loved ones, acquaintances, and coworkers. Maintaining and strengthening relationships requires consistent communication.

10. Diversify Your Network: Connect with people from all walks of life, occupations, and areas of expertise to broaden your network. A wide range of resources are available from a broad network.

While it's necessary to make connections with others, it's just as crucial to establish limits. 11. Establish your boundaries and make sure you can give your relationships the time and attention they deserve.

Stay upbeat and optimistic when meeting new people and developing professional connections. Optimism and a positive attitude might bring together a group of people who will encourage one another.

The Value of Social Support in Numerous Aspects of Your Life

The positive effects of having a strong social network extend to many facets of our lives. Let's investigate how networks can improve professional, personal, and communal development.

Personal 1.

   Emotional resilience is the capacity to bounce back from adversity and difficult circumstances with the help of one's social network.

   Friendships forged within these communities provide not only social support but also a feeling of shared experience and community.

   Improved mental health and lower rates of depression and anxiety have been related to social interactions.

   - Lifestyle Habits: Through shared activities and accountability, networks can impact lifestyle choices including exercise, good eating, and stress management.

Two: Professional:

- Professional Development: Making connections with other professionals can provide doors to internships, mentorships, and insider knowledge.

- Skill Development: Supportive networks offer possibilities for skill development, learning from others' experiences, and developing expertise.

- Job Satisfaction: A pleasant workplace with helpful coworkers is important to feeling fulfilled in one's employment.

- Collaboration: Collaboration and teamwork are increased within networks, leading to innovative problem-solving and invention.

Three, Community Involvement:

By bringing together people who care about the same things, supportive networks have a positive effect on society as a whole.

Volunteering, advocacy, and other forms of community improvement can all benefit from increased involvement with existing social networks.
Sharing resources, such as information, expertise, and material goods, is an important part of community life.
- Civic Engagement: Supportive networks can inspire civic participation and involvement in local or global issues.

Real-World Examples of Helpful Communities

The many ways in which social networks can improve the lives of their members and their communities are illustrated by the following examples drawn from real life.

Parents Seek Advice From Their Children's Teachers More Often Than Their Children Seek Advice From Their Teachers. Emotional support, parental advice, and a shared experience in childrearing are all things that can be found at parenting support groups.

In the corporate sector, professional networks like industry associations and networking events are crucial for advancing one's career, finding new employment, and forming new partnerships with one's peers.

3. Online Communities: Online communities, such as groups and forums on social media sites, bring together people from all over the world who share interests ranging from hobbies to careers.
4. Mentorship Programmes: Mentorship programmes in academia, business, and non-profit organisations provide guidance, coaching, and skill development for mentees.
Community organisations are a great way for neighbours to get together and work on neighbourhood issues, encourage participation in government, and enhance the quality of life for everyone.

6. Supportive Friendships: Close

Friendships developed over time provide invaluable emotional support, guidance, and companionship to its holders.

Conclusion

Building and maintaining supporting networks is a crucial part of human connection and well-being. Emotional wellness, personal development, and career achievement are all aided by having strong social networks. They cushion one's fall during hard times and improve one's quality of life in many ways.

Networking, providing assistance to others, seeking out mentors, and engaging in communities where one's interests and aspirations are shared are all ways in which people might grow their own webs of support. Personal, professional, and community spheres all benefit from having a strong network of people who have your back, making them an invaluable asset in overcoming adversity and realising one's potential. Investing in and nurturing meaningful relationships can provide for a richer and more satisfying life experience.

Chapter 7:
Mindfulness-Based Stress Reduction

7.1- The impact of stress on mental health

Psychological Effects of Stress

Work, relationships, money worries, and health issues are just some of the common sources of stress that people experience. Although some degree of stress is acceptable and even helpful, prolonged or extreme stress can have serious consequences for one's mental health. The impact of stress on the brain, its possible ramifications for a person's mental health, and methods for coping with and reducing stress are all topics we'll cover in this article.

Stress: An Overview

The "fight or flight" response is a frequent metaphor for the body's physiological reaction to stressful situations. Hormones such as cortisol and adrenaline are secreted by the body in response to stress, priming it to take action. Paraphrase includes heightened attentiveness and diverted energy resources. This higher heart rate includes increased energy resources.

While stress is adaptive in situations that necessitate quick action, such as escaping danger, it can become harmful when experienced chronically or excessively. Job demands, marital problems, financial difficulties, and health worries are just a few examples of the kinds of recurrent stresses that can add up over time and lead to chronic stress.

The Link Between Stress and Emotional Well-Being

The state of one's mind is directly related to their stress levels. There is a complex interplay between the two, with stress both causing and exacerbating mental health problems. Here are some basic ways stress effects mental health:

Anxiety disorders, number one:

Overwhelming anxiety, restlessness, and tension are hallmarks of Generalised Anxiety Disorder (GAD), and chronic stress is a major risk factor for this disorder.

The symptoms of panic disorder include sudden and acute bouts of terror or discomfort. Stress can induce panic attacks and increase the symptoms of panic disorder.

- Social Anxiety Disorder: Symptoms of social anxiety can be made worse by the stress of being among other people.

Depression (2):
The onset of depression is commonly linked to emotional or psychological stress. Repeated bouts of depression are also made more likely by chronic stress.

Stress can amplify depressive symptoms and hinder recovery, so it's important to keep that in mind.

PTSD (Post-Traumatic Stress Disorder): 3.

Flashbacks, nightmares, and extreme anxiety are all hallmarks of post-traumatic stress disorder (PTSD), which can develop after exposure to traumatic stressors including accidents, violence, or natural disasters.

- Chronic Stress: Prolonged exposure to stressful situations can exacerbate PTSD symptoms and make it harder to deal with painful memories.

Substance abuse, number four:

- Coping Mechanism: Substance addiction, including alcohol and drugs, is a coping mechanism for certain people. Addiction and mental health problems can also develop as a result of this.

Sleep disorders (5)
- Insomnia: Disrupted sleep patterns brought on by stress can exacerbate mood and brain function issues.

Cognitive Operation 6:

- Memory and Concentration: Chronic stress can impair memory and concentration, making it difficult to focus on tasks and accomplish them properly.

- Decision-Making: Stress can lead to poor decision-making and a tendency to dwell on negative thoughts and results.

7. Impact on Physical Health:

Physical health problems, such heart disease, gastrointestinal disorders, and chronic pain, are often companions to mental health concerns and stress.

Stress can make it more difficult for those with chronic illnesses to manage their symptoms.

Strategies to Manage and Mitigate Stress:

The detrimental effects of stress on mental health make it all the more important to develop methods of dealing with and reducing it. Some proven methods to alleviate stress and safeguard mental health are listed below.

First, Relaxation Methods and Mindfulness:

Focusing on the here and now, as in mindfulness meditation, has been shown to have positive effects on one's state of mind and anxiety levels.

The relaxation response in the body can be triggered by doing deep, diaphragmatic breathing exercises, which can also help reduce stress.

For example, you can practise progressive muscle relaxation by systematically tensing and relaxing different muscular groups.

Second, Physical Effort:

Regular exercise is an effective method for reducing stress and depression because it triggers the release of endorphins, the body's natural "feel-good" chemicals.

- Yoga: Yoga is a practise that blends physical postures, breathing exercises, and meditation to promote relaxation and decrease stress.
3. Make Healthier Decisions:
A well-balanced diet has been shown to improve mental wellness. Limit your intake of sugar and caffeine and focus instead on eating nutritious foods.

Adjusting to a new surroundings is not the same as adjusting to a new and more restful sleep environment.

Avoid excessive drinking and drug use because it can amplify the negative effects of stress and other mental health issues.

4. Social Support :

Keep in touch with those you care about and give them your undivided attention. Being among loved ones can ease loneliness and provide much-needed emotional support.Make an appointment with a therapist or counsellor if you feel you need extra support in dealing with stress or mental health issues.

5. Methods for Coping with Stress:

- Time Management: Set goals and make a plan to accomplish them in order to avoid becoming overwhelmed.
- Problem Solving: Take a proactive stance towards stressors. Dissect difficult tasks into more manageable chunks.Avoid placing undue pressure on yourself by striving for impossible outcomes, and be aware of the constraints you face. Self-care (number six)
Pursue interests and pastimes that make you happy and help you unwind.- Self-Compassion: Show yourself compassion and understanding when you're feeling overwhelmed. Keeping a notebook in which you write down your thoughts and feelings is a great way to deal with stress and gain perspective.

7 Expert Assistance:

Therapy and counselling can help you deal with the causes of your stress and develop healthy coping mechanisms.medicines: Managing mental health disorders made worse by stress may necessitate the use of medicines prescribed by a healthcare professional.

Conscious Technology Use 8.

Stress and anxiety can be caused by excessive technology use, which can be avoided by taking a vacation from screens and social media.

Use apps and online services aimed at relieving stress, increasing awareness, or calming the mind.

Practical Stress-Reduction Strategies

Examples from real life show how stress management can help safeguard mental health:

Yoga for Stress Reduction: 1.

As a means of dealing with the persistent anxiety brought on by their job, one person took up yoga. Practising yoga regularly has helped me calm down, concentrate better, and unwind.

2. Counselling and Peer Support:

A depressed person went to see a therapist and end up in a support group

group therapy or a support system. In treatment, they developed skills for dealing with stress, and in the support group, they found acceptance and friendship.

Alterations to One's Way of Life

An individual who was experiencing health problems as a result of stress made adjustments to their lifestyle by starting an exercise programme, switching to a healthier diet, and making getting enough sleep a higher priority. Because of these adjustments, they experienced a dramatic decrease in stress and an increase in general health.

Conclusion

Unavoidable as it is, stress can have serious effects on one's mental health. Anxiety, sadness, and post-traumatic stress disorder are just some of the mental health issues that can be exacerbated by prolonged or extreme stress. The first and most important step in protecting and improving mental health is learning to recognise the warning signals of stress and putting those lessons into practise.

Mindfulness and relaxation practises, a healthy lifestyle, social support, and, if necessary, professional help can all be effective ways for individuals to deal with stress. Real-world examples show that it is possible for people, with the correct tools and guidance, to effectively manage stress and protect their mental health, ultimately leading to a happier, healthier, and more fulfilled existence.

7.2- Mindfulness-based stress reduction techniques

Techniques for Reducing Stress Through Mindfulness

Stress is an inevitable part of life in today's fast-paced, high-stakes society. Whether it's due to job, relationships, health difficulties, or other things, stress may take a toll on our emotional and physical well-being. An approach that has been shown to effectively manage and reduce stress is called Mindfulness-Based Stress Reduction (MBSR). In this piece, we will delve into the core tenets of MBSR, as well as the different mindfulness practises it contains, and discuss how they can be used to alleviate stress, improve mental health, and encourage overall happiness.

Learning About MBSR (Mindfulness-Based Stress Reduction)

Dr. Jon Kabat-Zinn of the University of Massachusetts Medical Centre established the Mindfulness-Based Stress Reduction (MBSR) programme in the late 1970s. Stress, anxiety, and general well-being can all be better managed with this unique blend of yoga and meditation. The main principles of MBSR include:

To begin, there is Mindfulness Meditation:

- Present Moment Awareness: MBSR guides participants through the process of developing present moment awareness by encouraging them to observe their internal experiences without judgement.
Participants learn to notice their ideas without judgement or attachment, which sheds light on their underlying thought processes.

Paying attention to one's breathing, known as "mindful breathing," is one of the cornerstones of the Mindfulness-Based Stress Reduction (MBSR) programme.

Yoga and other forms of mindful movement (2):

   Yoga and other mindful movement exercises used in MBSR help increase awareness of one's body, leading to more flexibility and less stress in the body.

   Physical stress and discomfort can be reduced with the help of gentle yoga poses and stretching exercises.

Stress-Relieving Methods, Method No. 3:

   - Stress Response: MBSR provides individuals with the insight to understand their typical responses to stressful situations, as well as the resources to respond more effectively.

   Participants learn a variety of coping skills for dealing with stress in a healthy way.

Self-compassion 4.
   - Non-Judgment and Self-Acceptance: MBSR encourages people to treat themselves with kindness and understanding, which is a key component of self-compassion.

   - Emotional Regulation: Individuals learn to control their emotions, making it easier to deal with stressful feelings.

   MBSR's Mindfulness-Based Methods

The Mindfulness-Based Stress Reduction (MBSR) programme is a comprehensive set of methods for incorporating mindfulness into daily life. Relaxation and stress reduction are the byproducts of increased awareness of one's inner experiences gained through the practise of these methods. Some of the most important mindfulness practises often covered in MBSR include:

Scan the Body ():

The body scan is a mental exercise in which you focus on your physical feelings and any areas of tension or discomfort as you move from head to toe.

- Advantages: It helps you unwind, become more in tune with your body, and let go of stress in your muscles.

"Mindful Breathing" (2):
- Exercise: Pay attention to the breath by tracking its innate beat. Focus on the feeling of air going in and out of your lungs.

The practise of mindful breathing has many positive psychological and physiological effects.

Meditation in a Seated Position (3):

- Exercise: Sit in a position of comfort and focus on the here and now. Feel what you're feeling and think what you're thinking without passing judgement.

Benefits of sitting meditation include improved self-awareness, emotional regulation, and the capacity to respond to stressful situations rather than react to them.

Loving-Kindness Meditation (4):

Sending well-wishes and optimistic thoughts to oneself and others is a good practise. Begin with something simple like, "I pray that this day finds me happy, healthy, and at peace."

- Focus: - Focus: - Focus: The practise of meditation can help you feel more connected to others and to yourself.

5. Mindful Movement (Yoga):

Maintaining an awareness of your breath and your body as you perform mild yoga poses and movements is the practise.

- Advantages: Yoga and mindful movement increase mobility, lessen stress, and deepen the connection between body and mind.

Mindfulness in a Casual Setting 6.

- Exercise : Incorporate mindful awareness into routine tasks like eating, walking, and even dishwashing. Pay attention in the here and now, focusing on your senses.

- Advantages: Practising informal mindfulness might help you become more present and less reactive in your daily life.

Mindful Walking (7):

- Exercise: Strive to walk slowly and mindfully, focusing on the sensations of each step and your immediate surroundings.

The benefits of mindful walking include a greater understanding of how the body moves, decreased stress levels, and a deeper connection to nature.

Mindfulness-based stress reduction's (MBSR) advantages are numerous.
Extensive research on MBSR has shown that the practise has far-reaching advantages for mental and physical health. Notable advantages include:

Reducing Stress: 1.

By teaching people how to deal with stress in more constructive ways, MBSR can help lessen people's reactions to stressful situations.

Reducing Anxiety 2.

Through fostering emotional regulation and lessening rumination, the mindfulness techniques taught in MBSR have been shown to alleviate the symptoms of anxiety disorders.

Improved Mood 3.

- Practising mindfulness produces a more pleasant mood, more emotional balance, and increased general well-being.

Better Control of Emotions (4):

Participants in Mindfulness-Based Stress Reduction (MBSR) programmes report feeling more in command of their emotions and behaviour.

Better Sleep (5):

By encouraging relaxation and decreasing anxious thoughts, MBSR techniques can help people with insomnia get a better night's rest.

6. Greater Awareness of Oneself:

Insight into one's own mental processes and behavioural tendencies can be gained via the practise of mindfulness.

Better Focus (7):

Focus and concentration are improved with MBSR, which can help in many areas of life.

8. Improved Connections:

- Mindfulness approaches, such as loving-kindness meditation, can promote empathy, compassion, and interpersonal connections.

Pain Management (9):

Individuals with chronic pain issues can benefit from utilising MBSR as part of a pain treatment programme.
General Happiness (10):

MBSR improves health and happiness by teaching people how to relax and focus their attention inward.

Advantages of MBSR in Practise

Some real-world examples of MBSR's life-altering effects are as follows:

Reducing Workplace Stress: 1.

An individual with job-related stress and burnout decided to participate in a Mindfulness-Based Stress Reduction (MBSR) course. They improved their health and happiness at work by learning to deal with stress in healthier ways through the practise of mindfulness.

Dealing with Anxiety:

Someone with generalised anxiety disorder (GAD) started doing mindfulness meditation every day. They felt less anxious and stressed out over time and were better able to control their emotions.

Management of Chronic Pain:
A person who suffers from chronic

pain took part in a Mindfulness-Based Stress Reduction (MBSR) course. They found that practising mindfulness helped them deal with the emotional and physical strain of their discomfort.

Conclusion

The Mindfulness-Based Stress Reduction (MBSR) programme is an effective method of stress management and reduction that has been shown to improve both mental and physical health. Practical methods for developing present-moment awareness, better self-regulation, and emotional well-being are provided by the tenets of mindfulness meditation, yoga, and stress reduction approaches.

The numerous mindfulness techniques within MBSR, such as the body scan, mindful breathing, and loving-kindness meditation, can be integrated into daily life to promote relaxation, reduce anxiety, and enhance overall quality of life. From decreased stress to enhanced emotional control and a more general sense of well-being, real-world examples show how MBSR may make a difference in people's lives. Individuals can begin a journey towards greater inner calm and resilience in the face of life's hardships by adopting these practises.

7.3- Creating a mindful daily routine

How to Build a Conscious Habitual Practise

It's simple to become stressed out by life's constant demands in today's fast-paced society. The constant flow of information and distractions, on top of our regular work and family obligations, can easily overwhelm and disengage us. However, by practising mindfulness on a regular basis, we can achieve better self-awareness, emotional stability, and mental peace. In this piece, we'll talk about the value of developing a regular mindfulness practise, some easy ways to get started, and the numerous advantages it may bring to your mental and emotional health.

The Value of Maintaining a Conscious Daily Habit

Our everyday routine consists of repetitive actions that we carry out without giving them much attention. These habits affect how we invest our time and effort, which in turn can have far-reaching effects on our health. A mindful daily routine, in contrast, is one that is consciously structured to cultivate attention and present in each moment. Keeping a mindful practise as part of your daily life is crucial for several reasons.

Reducing Stress: 1.
   Practising mindfulness each day can help you find brief respites from your hectic schedule. Meditation and other forms of mindfulness training help people calm their minds and control their feelings. Newfound Consciousness 2.

   Mindfulness is the practise of bringing one's attention to one's internal experiences, such as one's thoughts, feelings, and bodily sensations, on a regular basis. Improved self-awareness and EQ are possible outcomes of this heightened sensitivity.

3. Enhanced Concentration and Efficiency:

Concentration and mental acuity can be improved by mindfulness practises like meditation and deep breathing. This has the potential to improve our efficiency and effectiveness in carrying out our duties.

Improved Connections (4):

The quality of our relationships with others can be enhanced by cultivating greater awareness and compassion. It frees us to give our undivided attention to the people we care about most.

Better Health, 5:

The immune system's ability to fight off disease is directly tied to the body's ability to fight off infection. A mindful daily habit can contribute to these health benefits.

"Emotional Resilience" (6):
Mindfulness training helps strengthen our emotional fortitude, allowing us to face adversity with more composure and less emotional outburst.

Practical Strategies for Creating a Mindful Daily Routine

Building a practise that incorporates mindfulness into your day-to-day activities takes time, effort, and a willingness to practise. Here are some doable methods for incorporating mindfulness into your daily life:

Mindfulness in the Morning :

Make a point to start your day off right by engaging in some form of morning mindfulness practise. Meditation, deep breathing, or just taking a few moments to think on what you're grateful for are all good examples.

Mindful Eating (2):

Eat gently, focus on the flavours and textures, and savour each bite as part of a mindful eating practise. You should not eat while watching TV or working.

"Mindful Movement" (No. 3):
Yoga, stretching, and mindful walks are all great ways to include movement into your daily routine. Focus on your breathing and internal sensations as you move.

4. Recesses:

Plan periodic checks in with yourself throughout the day. Take some deep breaths, stretch, or just be in the moment during these pauses.

Mindful Work (5):

Integrate meditation or mindful awareness into your workday by taking brief breaks to focus on your breathing. This can help relieve stress and boost productivity.

Digital detox (6):

Disconnect from screens and gadgets at regular intervals. Put up barriers to keep digital distractions at bay and your focused moments intact.

Mindful Transitions (7):

- Approach transitions between activities with mindfulness. Before beginning a new activity, such as leaving work, starting a meeting, or entering your home, take a few deep breaths.

8 Thoughts for the Evening:

Do some quick thinking as you wind down for the night. Think about your day with genuine interest and kindness towards yourself. Think about the good and the bad, and where you may use some tweaks.

9. Gratitude Practise:

Start a thankfulness diary and write down three things every day that you're thankful for. By doing this, you may train your mind to concentrate on the bright side of things.

Mindful Evening Routine (10):

Create a winding down and mindful nighttime ritual. Reading, light stretching, and a relaxing soak in a hot tub are all good examples.

The Value of a Conscious Daily Routine

The positive effects of incorporating mindfulness into your everyday routine are far-reaching and can improve many facets of your existence. Some of the good things that could happen are listed below.

Reducing Stress: 1.

Including meditation or other mindfulness practises into your everyday life has been shown to improve mental health and well-being.

Controlling one's emotions:

Mindfulness can help you improve your ability to control your emotions and react to adversity with more composure since it raises your level of self-awareness.

3. Enhanced Concentration and Efficiency:

Mindfulness-based interventions have been shown to increase attention and cognition, leading to greater efficiency in many areas of life.

Improved Connections (4):

- Mindfulness encourages greater communication, empathy, and presence, which can improve the quality of your interactions with loved ones.

Better Health, 5:

Lower blood pressure, less inflammation, and stronger immunity are just some of the physical benefits linked to practising mindfulness.

"Emotional Resilience" (6):

Including mindfulness meditation into your daily routine might help you become more emotionally resilient and cope better with life's difficulties.

Practical Illustrations of Mindful Habits
Examples from everyday life show how the transformative impacts of mindfulness may be experienced by anyone, anywhere.

The Morning Meditation Routine:

A daily practise of ten minutes of meditation to set an optimistic tone for the day. They utilise it to keep their nerves in check and their minds on the job.

Mindful Eating: 2.

A family sits down to a peaceful meal together. They eat slowly, talk about the best parts of their day, and enjoy every bite.

3. Work Breaks for Mindfulness:

A busy office worker takes periodic breaks to focus on his or her breathing and engage in other mindfulness practises. This method has been shown to be effective in reducing stress and promoting concentration.

Evening Mindfulness Practise:

Reading, keeping a journal, and light stretching become regular parts of one's nightly routine. They will be more relaxed and ready for a good night's sleep thanks to this practise.
Conclusion

Even with all the stresses and distractions of modern life, a regular practise of mindfulness can do wonders for one's mental and emotional health. Mindfulness is a practise that can help you become more present in the moment, better able to control your emotions, and generally less stressed. You may improve your overall sense of well-being and happiness by implementing the suggestions presented here into your everyday routine. Mindfulness is a gift you give yourself; it helps you deal with the ups and downs of life with more grace and fortitude.

Chapter 8:
Using Meditation to Recover from Trauma

8.1- Understanding trauma and its effects
The Consequences of Trauma, Comprehended

Traumatization is a traumatic experience that can have long-lasting and far-reaching impacts on individuals. Many different things, from physical harm to mental anguish, might trigger this condition. In this post, we will investigate what trauma is, how it manifests itself, and the wide-ranging consequences it can have for a person's mental, emotional, and physical health.

Determining What Trauma Is

A traumatic experience is one that is so upsetting that it overwhelms a person's coping mechanisms and leaves permanent emotional, psychological, or bodily scars. Fear, helplessness, or dread are common reactions to its onset, which may be sudden or gradual. What one person considers traumatic may not be the same as what another considers horrific.

The following are some broad categories into which various forms of trauma can be placed:

Injury to the body: 1.

Accidents, falls, and violent attacks all qualify as examples of physical trauma. Long-term impairment concerns might lead to long-term suffering.

(2) Psychological or Emotional Trauma:

Distressing experiences that have an adverse effect on a person's mental and emotional health can lead to what is known as emotional or psychological trauma. Examples include emotional abuse, betrayal, or witnessing a tragic occurrence.

Trauma in Early Development (3):

Neglect, abuse, or a broken bond to parents can all cause developmental trauma in children. The ability to control one's emotions and maintain healthy relationships can be permanently damaged.

Complex Trauma, Number Four:

Multi- or long-term exposure to interpersonal trauma is a hallmark of complex trauma. Complex post-traumatic stress disorder (C-PTSD) is just one of the mental health issues that might result.

Secondary Trauma: 5. Secondary Traumatic Exposure: 5.

Secondary trauma, often called vicarious trauma or compassion fatigue, happens when people, such as healthcare workers, first responders, or carers, are exposed to the painful experiences of others.

Trauma's Aftermath

The psychological, emotional, and physiological health of a person can be severely compromised by traumatic experiences. These outcomes may have far-reaching consequences and might show themselves in a variety of forms. Some of the most common reactions to trauma are:

1. Post-Traumatic Stress Disorder (PTSD):

Exposure to a traumatic event can result in the development of post-traumatic stress disorder (PTSD). Flashbacks, nightmares, extreme anxiety, and heightened vigilance are all possible symptoms.

The Anxiety

Depression and other anxiety disorders have a strong link to traumatic experiences. It can cause you to feel down and out and hopeless and anxious all the time.

3. Dissociation:

Dissociation is a coping technique wherein victims of trauma separate themselves from their own thoughts, feelings, and environments. It can cause a person to feel alienated from their own identity.

Emotional Dysregulation: 4.

Mood swings, explosive anger, and an inability to deal with stress are just some of the emotional difficulties that can result from experiencing trauma.

5. Difficulties With Self-Esteem:

- Shame, guilt, and a generally negative sense of one's own worth are common outcomes of traumatic experiences.

6. Difficulties in Relationships:

Relational health can be harmed by traumatic experiences. It may lead to trust concerns, social isolation, or difficulty in building attachments.

7. Substance Abuse:

- Some individuals turn to drugs or alcohol as a way to cope with the emotional agony of trauma, leading to substance misuse difficulties.

8. Physical Health Problems:

   - Trauma can contribute to a number of physical health concerns, including chronic pain, gastrointestinal disorders, and cardiovascular disease.

9. Sleep Disturbances:

   - Trauma typically leads to sleep difficulties, such as sleeplessness, nightmares, and night sweats.

10. Impact on Daily Functioning:

   A person's capacity to engage in everyday activities, such as job, school, and social interactions, might be negatively impacted by traumatic experiences.

Complex Trauma and C-PTSD

Complex trauma, as described previously, entails exposure to several or extended traumatic events, frequently within interpersonal interactions. It can develop in a condition known as complex post-traumatic stress disorder (C-PTSD). C-PTSD is characterized by symptoms that go beyond those normally linked with PTSD. Some of the primary features of C-PTSD include:

1. Emotional Dysregulation:

   - Individuals with C-PTSD may struggle with powerful and fast changing emotions, making it tough to manage their moods.

2. Disturbances in Self-Identity:

   - C-PTSD can lead to a fragmented sense of self, with individuals feeling estranged from their identity and values.

3. Difficulties in Relationships:

   - People with C-PTSD generally find challenges in creating and maintaining good relationships, which can contribute to a sense of isolation.

4. Chronic Feelings of Shame and Guilt:

   Self-loathing and guilt are common symptoms of C-PTSD, and they can be quite debilitating.

Somatic Symptoms (5):

   Physical symptoms, such as chronic pain, gastrointestinal problems, and other somatic complaints, are a possible manifestation of C-PTSD.

Coping with Trauma and Seeking Help

Coping with trauma is a complex and individualised process, and healing can differ from person to person. However, reaching out for assistance is essential for recovery. Important factors to think about when overcoming trauma are as follows:

1. Therapy and Counselling:

   Trauma-focused psychotherapies, such as cognitive-behavioral therapy (CBT) and eye movement desensitisation and reprocessing

(EMDR), have been shown to be particularly useful in alleviating the symptoms of post-traumatic stress disorder (PTSD).

Medication (2):

Depression-------------------- Medications are sometimes used to treat symptoms of depression or anxiety.

Supportive Relationships 3.

Communicating with those who care about you might help you feel accepted and validated on a deep emotional level.

Self-Care 4.

Self-care practises including mindfulness, physical activity, and relaxation techniques can aid survivors in coping with the mental and physical after-effects of trauma.

Groups for social and emotional support (5)

A sense of understanding and mutual healing can be found in communities or support groups of people who have endured similar traumas.

Security and Limits (6):
Creating and upholding safe spaces and limits is crucial for trauma survivors. This could mean avoiding the culprit as much as possible or making the area where you are more secure.
7. Constructing Resilience:

Individuals can better manage the difficulties of healing from trauma if they practise resilience-building activities like mindfulness, meditation, and self-compassion.

8. Expert Assistance:

Consulting with mental health specialists who have experience working with trauma survivors helps equip victims with the knowledge and resources they need to heal.

Conclusion

Understanding trauma and its

We're talking about the psychological and mental well-being of people here, as well as the obvious physical health and fitness benefits. It's important to get help after experiencing trauma because the repercussions can linger for a long time if they aren't handled. Recognising the signs of trauma and seeking help are critical steps towards healing and recovery.

Keep in mind that recovery from trauma is doable, and that helpful treatments and resources are out there. Individuals can reclaim their life' sense of control, resilience, and well-being with the help of appropriate resources and a dedication to the recovery process.

8.2- Mindfulness as a tool for healing trauma

Healing Trauma with Mindfulness

A traumatic event is extremely upsetting and can have long-term effects on a person's psychological, emotional, and physiological health. Trauma, whether caused by a single traumatic incident or by chronic exposure to stressful conditions, can have severe consequences. Fortunately, mindfulness has become a highly effective method for dealing with trauma and facilitating recovery. In this post, we'll look into how mindfulness relates to trauma, how it can help with healing, and how to include it into the process of getting over traumatic experiences.

The of Trauma and Its Effects on Mental Health.

It's important to learn about what trauma is and how it affects people before trying to use mindfulness as a treatment for it. The following are some examples of traumatic experiences:

Accidents, traumas, and invasive medical procedures all qualify as examples of physical trauma.
- Psychological or emotional trauma: caused by experiences such as abuse, neglect, or exposure to traumatic events.
- Developmental Trauma: affecting a child's development, typically through attachment disturbances or persistently negative experiences.
Involving multiple or protracted exposure to traumatic experiences, typically within social contexts. - Complex Trauma.
Secondary trauma occurs in people like healthcare workers and first responders who are exposed to the terrible experiences of others.

The repercussions of trauma can be substantial and may emerge in numerous ways, including:

Flashbacks, nightmares, extreme anxiety, and hyperawareness are all hallmarks of Post-Traumatic Stress Disorder (PTSD).
Trauma is a major contributor to the development of both mood and anxiety disorders.
Dissociation is a coping strategy in which one becomes emotionally or mentally detached from one's current situation.
- Emotional Dysregulation: the inability to control and moderate one's feelings, as seen by erratic behaviour and explosive rage.
- Self-Esteem Issues: Often leading in emotions of shame, guilt, and a negative self-image.
Difficulty in creating and sustaining healthy partnerships. Difficulty in forming and keeping healthy relationships.
- Substance Abuse: Some people abuse drugs or alcohol to numb the emotional agony they feel after experiencing trauma.
Conditions of the body, such as persistent discomfort, digestive problems, and heart disease.

The effects of trauma on one's health can be far-reaching and long-lasting. However, mindfulness offers a road to healing and rehabilitation.

The Benefits of Mindfulness for Post-Traumatic Growth

Mindfulness is a set of skills that emphasises paying attention in the here and now without passing judgement or analysing one's experiences. It's a practise that helps people be more in the moment, whether it's with internal or external stimuli. Practising mindfulness encourages an openness and lack of judgement towards one's internal and external events. Because of these benefits, mindfulness is an effective method for dealing with trauma:

1. Reducing the Impact of Intrusive Thoughts and Memories: 1. Reducing the Impact of Intrusive Thoughts

Intrusive memories and thoughts are a common result of traumatic experiences. Meditation and other forms of mindfulness training help people become more objective observers of their thoughts and feelings, allowing them to pass more quickly and with less impact.

Improving Control Over Emotions 2.

Emotional intelligence and control can be developed through practising mindfulness. By gaining the capacity to perceive emotions without becoming overwhelmed, individuals can better regulate and cope with overwhelming feelings linked with trauma.

3: Establishing Stability and Security

Disconnection and a heightened sense of vulnerability are common reactions to trauma. Practising mindfulness can give you a firm footing in the here and now, which can help you feel more secure and at ease.

4. Learning to Be Kind to Yourself:

Self-blame and low self-esteem are common issues for people who have survived traumatic experiences. Self-compassion is fostered through cultivating a mindful perspective that is kind and accepting of oneself.

Five, Building Resilience to Adversity:

Mindfulness trains people to stay with unpleasant feelings rather than running away or using unhealthy coping techniques. In the case of trauma recovery, this is a crucial asset.

Resilience and post-traumatic growth promotion:

- Mindfulness can help individuals develop resilience and ultimately find meaning and growth in the aftermath of trauma. The ability to bounce back from setbacks is honed.

Improving Relationships with Others:

Better understanding and interaction between people is made possible by cultivating mindfulness. Those who have been through emotional or relational trauma should pay extra attention to this.

Useful Mindfulness-Based Strategies for Trauma Recovery

Regular practise of mindfulness techniques is essential for incorporating mindfulness into the process of recovering from trauma. These methods aid in the cultivation of knowledge and abilities crucial for overcoming obstacles encountered during the healing process from traumatic experiences. Some helpful mindfulness practises for post-traumatic growth are as follows:

Mindful Breathing (1):

Maintain a mindful awareness of your breathing. Feel how your lungs expand and contract as you breathe in and out. The mind wanders, and you gently bring it back to its original focus.

breath.

Second, a Body Scan:

Scan your body from head to toe, mentally taking stock of how everything is going. Take note of how you feel and pinpoint any areas of stress.

3. Mindful Meditation:

Maintain a daily meditation practise in which you concentrate on your breathing, your body, or a mantra. Meditation helps develop a sense of inner serenity and clarity.

4. Grounding Techniques:

Reconnect with your immediate surroundings and take your mind off of upsetting thoughts or memories with grounding techniques like the 5-4-3-2-1 exercise.

5. Loving-Kindness Meditation:

Sending positive thoughts and feelings to oneself and others is a key component of loving-kindness meditation. This can foster self-compassion and empathy.

6. Mindful Movement:

- Engage in mindful movement practices like yoga or tai chi. Pay attention to your breath and the sensations in your body as you move.

7. Journaling:

- Keep a mindfulness journal to record your thoughts, emotions, and experiences. Journaling can provide insight into your trauma-related patterns and progress.

8. Mindful Walking:

- Take mindful walks in nature or around your neighborhood. Pay attention to each step, your surroundings, and the sensations of walking.

9. Sensory Mindfulness:

- Engage your senses mindfully. Notice the sights, sounds, tastes, smells, and textures of your surroundings.

10. Compassion for Self and Others:

   - Practice self-compassion by treating yourself with the same care and understanding you would provide to a friend. Extend this kindness to others as well.

Real-Life Examples of Mindfulness in Trauma Healing

Real-life examples highlight the impact of mindfulness on trauma healing:

1. PTSD Recovery:

   - An individual with PTSD uses mindfulness meditation into their everyday regimen. Over time, they report reduced symptoms, including fewer flashbacks and nightmares.

Controlling one's emotions:

   - Someone who endured emotional trauma employs mindfulness techniques to improve emotional regulation. They discover that they can regulate intense emotions more successfully and respond to triggers with greater equanimity.

3. Relationship Healing:

   - A victim of relational trauma participates in a mindfulness-based group treatment program. Through mindfulness practices, they build healthier patterns of communication and connection in their relationships.

Conclusion

Trauma is a difficult and stressful experience that can have far-reaching impacts on individuals' lives. The road of healing trauma typically involves multidimensional assistance, and mindfulness is a powerful tool that can facilitate recovery. By promoting present-moment awareness, emotional control, self-compassion, and resilience, mindfulness practices help individuals to negotiate the challenges of trauma healing with greater ease and inner strength.

It's vital to remember that healing from trauma is a unique and individual process, and mindfulness is one of many solutions accessible. Seeking professional treatment from therapists and mental health experts who specialize in trauma is frequently a vital step in the recovery journey. With the integration of mindfulness practises and therapeutic assistance, individuals can proceed toward a path of healing, resilience, and post-traumatic growth.

8.3- Therapeutic approaches combining mindfulness and trauma recovery

Integrating Mindfulness-Based Therapy into Posttraumatic Growth

Because traumatic experiences can have far-reaching impacts, the process of recovering from them can be lengthy and difficult. Fortunately, therapeutic approaches have arisen that combine mindfulness and trauma recovery, and these skills can greatly assist survivors on their road to healing and resilience. This article will discuss the benefits of mindfulness-based therapies for trauma survivors, as well as the ways in which mindfulness can aid in healing from trauma.

The Intersection of Mindfulness and Trauma Recovery

Mindfulness is a form of contemplative practise that emphasises paying attention in the present moment, keeping an open mind, and showing kindness to oneself. It helps people to take in everything going on around them, from their thoughts and feelings to their bodily sensations and environmental cues. Due to its ability to assist trauma survivors deal with the upsetting and often overwhelming repercussions of trauma, mindfulness is a perfect fit for trauma rehabilitation.

Trauma recovery, on the other hand, is a process of healing and restoring a sense of safety, self-worth, and empowerment after experiencing trauma. The emotional, psychological, and physical wounds of trauma must be healed in this process, and resilience and post-traumatic growth must be fostered.

There are several critical areas where mindfulness and trauma rehabilitation meet:

1) Emotional Self-Control:

Practising mindfulness can help trauma survivors learn to control their emotions, making it easier for them to deal with painful feelings without succumbing to them. Those suffering from emotional dysregulation as a result of trauma will find this to be of great use.

Self-Compassion: 2.

Self-compassion, fostered by mindfulness, is an effective antidote to the self-criticism and guilt that frequently accompany traumatic experiences. Those who make it through are the ones who learn to treat themselves with the same compassion and empathy they would show a friend.

Safety and Grounding 3.

Feelings of isolation and helplessness are common after experiencing trauma. Practising mindfulness can give you a firm footing in the here and now, which can help you feel more secure and at ease.

4. Post-Traumatic Growth and Resilience:

Mindfulness helps trauma survivors recover emotionally and spiritually so that they may move forward with their lives. It promotes a flexible approach to hardship.

Fifthly, Immunity to Trauma Triggers:

With the cultivation of a nonreactive awareness that mindfulness provides, individuals are better able to respond appropriately to trauma triggers. This decreases the emotional charge linked with painful memories and events.

Mindfulness-Based Trauma-Recovery Treatments

Mindfulness training is a crucial part of the healing process after trauma and is used in a variety of treatment approaches. These methods use the benefits of mindfulness to aid in the recovery process for those who have experienced trauma. Some of the most well-known therapy methods that incorporate mindfulness and trauma recovery are as follows:

1. Mindfulness-Based Stress Reduction (MBSR):

   - Developed by Dr. Jon Kabat-Zinn, MBSR is an evidence-based programme that incorporates mindfulness meditation, yoga, and stress reduction practises. In order to help those who have experienced trauma, the environment has been modified to reduce reactivity and promote emotional regulation.

"Mindfulness-Based Cognitive Therapy" (MBCT) is a " 2."

   Mindfulness-based cognitive therapy (MBCT) integrates mindfulness practises with cognitive-behavioral therapy (CBT). Trauma survivors benefit from it because it encourages them to be mindful of the here and now while also teaching them to recognise and reframe harmful thought patterns.

Dialectical behaviour therapy (DBT) is the third option.

   Mindfulness is one of the four pillars of Dr. Marsha Linehan's Dialectical Behaviour Therapy (DBT). Because CBT teaches people how to control their emotions and cope with distress, it is especially helpful for those suffering from trauma-related symptoms.

Eye-movement desensitisation and reprocessing (EMDR) is a 4

   For trauma treatment, nothing beats Eye Movement Desensitisation and Reprocessing (EMDR). Mindfulness is not a central tenet of this approach, but it is used at specific stages of treatment to aid in the processing of painful memories and the alleviation of discomfort.

5. Trauma-Informed Yoga:

Understanding the effects of trauma on the body with the benefits of yoga to create a holistic approach to healing. Its primary goals are to encourage self-control, a sense of stability, and personal agency.

Mindful Self-Compassion (MSC) (No. 6):

MSC is a self-compassion training programme created by psychologists Drs. Kristin Neff and Christopher Germer. It aids trauma survivors in developing more self-compassion and less self-criticism.

7 Compassion-Focused Therapy (CFT):

Developed by Dr. Paul Gilbert, CFT uses mindfulness and self-compassion strategies to counteract the feelings of guilt and blame that frequently follow traumatic experiences. It encourages kind thoughts and feelings within oneself.

Somatic Experiencing (SE) is a 8.

The trauma-body connection is at the heart of Dr. Peter A. Levine's somatic experiencing approach (SE). It combines paying attention to physiological feelings as a means of strengthening recovery and resiliency.

Benefits of Mindfulness-Based Trauma Therapy

Recovery

Several significant advantages accrue to trauma survivors when mindfulness is incorporated into the healing process:

1) Emotional Self-Control:

Paradoxically, fostering receptiveness and serenity in the face of adversity aids individuals with stronger emotional regulation and resiliency.

Lessened Sensitivity to Post-Traumatic Triggers:

The emotional weight of traumatic memories and experiences is lessened as survivors develop the ability to recognise trauma triggers without becoming overwhelmed by them.

3. Enhanced Self-Compassion:

Self-compassion, fostered by mindfulness, is an effective antidote to the self-criticism and guilt that frequently accompany traumatic experiences.

Increased fortitude 4:

Mindfulness helps survivors of trauma find meaning and growth by fostering resilience.

5. Enhanced Coping Capacity:

Better coping skills are learned, and unhealthy coping strategies like avoidance are abandoned.

Empowerment and Agency (6):

Practising mindfulness can help trauma survivors feel more in charge of their life by fostering a sense of agency and empowerment.

Quality of Life Improvements 7:

- Overall, mindfulness-informed trauma healing can lead to an enhanced quality of life, with individuals enjoying increased well-being and a stronger connection to themselves and others.

Case Studies of Mindfulness-Based Trauma Therapy

Real-life examples show the impact of mindfulness-informed trauma recovery:

PTSD Recovery with MBCT: 1.

Mindfulness-Based Cognitive Therapy (MBCT) is practised by a person who has undergone trauma. The intensity of their PTSD symptoms lessens when patients learn to detach themselves emotionally from their traumatic recollections through the use of mindfulness practises.

The Mindfulness Integration EMDR Protocol:

Eye Movement Desensitisation and Reprocessing (EMDR) therapy with mindfulness techniques is provided to an accident survivor. This method aids the survivor in working through difficult emotions and memories.

Yoga for Trauma Recovery:

A victim of childhood abuse takes part in rehabilitative yoga courses. They are able to improve their ability to self-regulate and let go of pent-up tension as a result of this practise.

Conclusion

Recovering from trauma is an individual and difficult process, but therapy techniques that integrate mindfulness and trauma recovery show promise as a way forward. By combining mindfulness practises into trauma therapy, individuals can acquire emotional regulation, self-compassion, and coping skills, ultimately leading to a higher sense of empowerment and well-being.

Each survivor's approach to the healing process is different, and the therapeutic method taken to each survivor's needs is different. Mindfulness can be a helpful addition to standard trauma therapy, and seeking the guidance of mental health specialists who specialise in trauma is frequently an essential step in the healing journey. Paradigm shift and post-trauma growth. Post-trauma shift and self-discovery. Self-discovery and post-trauma growth.

Chapter 9:
The Effects of Mindfulness on Individuals' Psychological Health

9.1- Mindfulness for children and adolescents

Meditation Training for Young People

Once thought of as a technique only useful for adults, mindfulness has recently been recognised for its potential to improve the lives of young people. Stress, anxiety, attention difficulties, and emotional control are just some of the issues that young people in today's fast-paced, digitally-connected society encounter. Mindfulness offers a range of benefits for children and adolescents, from improved mental health to enhanced academic achievement. In this post, we'll look at why mindfulness is so crucial for young people, how it may be used in schools, how to effectively teach it to kids and teens, and what good results they can expect to see.

Young People and the Benefits of Mindfulness

The mental and emotional health of today's children and teenagers is threatened by a variety of factors. Feelings of overload, anxiety, and distraction are common in today's society due to several factors, including academic expectations, social interactions, family issues, and the ubiquitous presence of digital devices. Youth can benefit greatly from mindfulness practises in overcoming these obstacles. Some of the many benefits of mindfulness for young people are listed below.

Reducing Stress: 1.

Mindfulness is a useful tool for stress management because it teaches young people to focus on the here-and-now rather than dwelling on the past or the future.

Controlling one's emotions:

Children and teenagers who engage in mindfulness practises have a stronger capacity for self-awareness and emotional regulation.

3 Increased Focus and Concentration:

- Mindfulness activities increase attention and focus, which can benefit students' academic performance and daily duties.

Awareness of Self-Awareness: Awareness of Self-Awareness of Self-Awareness of Self-A

Increased self-awareness and acceptance are the results for young people who take the time to learn about themselves and how they think.

Improved abilities to interact with others 5.

- Mindfulness improves empathy, compassion, and efficient communication, which are necessary for good interactions with peers and adults.

Lessening of Depressive and Anxious Symptoms (6):

Evidence suggests that practising mindfulness can help alleviate anxiety and despair in young people.

Enhanced Resilience 7.

The ability to recover from setbacks and hardships is enhanced via the practise of mindfulness.

Better Sleep Quality 8:

Meditation and other forms of mindfulness training have been shown to enhance sleep quality, which in turn benefits health and well-being.

The Role of Mindfulness in the Classroom

Mindfulness instruction for kids and teens should ideally take place in a school setting. Mindfulness-based interventions have been widely adopted by schools and universities as a means to improve students' health and academic performance. In schools, mindfulness is used in the following ways:

"Mindful Classroom Practises" () 1.

Teachers help their pupils unwind and concentrate by incorporating brief mindfulness activities into the everyday routine. These may include mindful breathing or guided meditations.

Mindful (2) Movement:

Yoga and tai chi are only two examples of the kind of mindful movement practises that are being included in some schools to promote students' overall health and happiness.

"Social and Emotional Learning" (SEL) is the third component.

To help students develop their EQ, EQi, and IPS, SEL programmes frequently incorporate mindfulness practises.

Resolution of Conflict:

- Mindfulness practises are used to teach conflict resolution and emotional regulation, helping students handle disagreements and challenges more effectively.

5. Test and Exam Anxiety Reduction:

Exam and test anxiety can be mitigated via the practise of mindfulness, allowing students to give their best performance even when the stakes are highest.

6. Preventing Bullying:

Empathy and kindness, fostered by mindfulness programmes, can help schools combat bullying.

Real-World Methods for Instilling Mindfulness in Young People

Young kids should be taught mindfulness using methods that are both age-appropriate and interesting to them. Some tried-and-true approaches to teaching mindfulness to kids and teens are outlined below.

1. Exercises for Improving Breathing:

It's important to instruct young people on basic breathing techniques, such as "breathing in for a count of four, holding for a count of four, and exhaling for a count of four." This can aid them in controlling their feelings and relieving tension.

Mindful Colouring (2):

Give your kids complex colouring pages and suggest they colour while focusing on the experience of the colours and the sensations they're having.

Three, Guided Imagery:

Guide children and teens through relaxing mental imagery exercises to help them unwind and cope with stressful situations.

4. Body Scan:

- Guide students through a body scan activity, urging them to focus on each part of their body, detecting feelings and releasing tension.

Mindful Listening (5):

Encourage students to practise attentive listening by having them listen to and reflect on various noises, such as those found in nature or the ringing of a bell.

Mindful Eating (6):

Teach your students the benefits of eating consciously by getting them to focus on the food's flavour, texture, and aroma while they consume it.

Journalists, 7:

Give your pupils diaries to record their innermost feelings and reflections. Encourage introspection and free expression through journaling.The Eighth Practise of Mindful Movement

– Incorporate meditative

yoga, stretching, and dance into after-school and school-based physical activity programmes.

Exercises of Gratitude 9.

- Encourage kids to practise thankfulness by writing down things they are glad for each day or sharing them with their peers.

Mindful games and apps are the tenth .

To make mindfulness practise more interesting and enjoyable for kids and teens, use games and apps made for that age group.

The Beneficial Effects of Mindfulness on Young People

There is a wide range of benefits associated with incorporating mindfulness practises into the lives of children and adolescents:

1. Better Academic Results:

Students who practise mindfulness report increased focus and fewer distractions in the classroom.

Increased Capacity for Emotional Self-Control

Young people can learn to control their feelings and curb irrational outbursts.

Improved Capacity to Bounce Back

Students who practise mindfulness are more likely to recover quickly from setbacks and difficulties.

4. Decreased Worry and Stress:

- Mindfulness practises help decrease symptoms of worry and tension, giving relief for pupils.

More empathy and compassion (5):

Young people increase their capacity for empathy and compassion, which promotes healthy connections and friendships.

Higher Quality Sleep (6):

Better sleep at night means more energy and concentration during the day.

Changes in Positive Behaviour 7.

Students generally demonstrate greater hostility. Paraphrase often exhibits increased collaboration.

8. Raised Confidence Levels:

Increased introspection and acceptance of oneself are direct results of practising mindfulness.

Examples of Actual Achievement

Real-life examples show the transforming effect of mindfulness for children and adolescents:

Improved Concentration and Stamina 1.

Daily breathing exercises and mindful listening are only two components of a new mindfulness programme at a middle school. According to their teachers, pupils are more focused and resilient in the face of academic challenges.

(2) Emotional Control:

A high school's social-emotional learning programme now includes mindfulness exercises. As a result, students report feeling more equipped to manage their emotions and handle disagreements efficiently.

Reduced Test Anxiety: 3

High school students practise mindfulness to calm their nerves before exams. They said they were more relaxed and assured while taking their tests as a result.

Conclusion

Teenagers and young adults can benefit much from practising mindfulness in today's fast-paced, always-connected environment. Mindfulness practises equip young people with increased resilience and well-being through fostering stress reduction, emotional control, improved attention, and enhanced social skills. Mindfulness may help children and teenagers in profound ways, both in and out of the classroom, laying the groundwork for happier, healthier lives in the years to come.

9.2- Mindfulness in older adults

Meditation and Ageing

The ancient practise of mindfulness, which is built on paying attention in the here and now, has recently been recognised for its potential to improve the quality of life for people of advanced age. Health issues, the death of loved ones, and philosophical doubts about the later phases of life are just some of the stressors that older people encounter in a society characterised by rapid change and the challenges of ageing. The practise of mindfulness has been shown to have numerous positive effects on the health, happiness, and longevity of those of retirement age. In this article, we will discuss the significance of mindfulness for older persons, its applicability in treating age-related difficulties, practical ways for bringing mindfulness into daily life, and the beneficial effects it can yield.

The Importance of Mindfulness in Ageing

Physical, mental, and interpersonal difficulties arise specifically for the elderly. Examples of such difficulties include:

- Physical Health Issues: such as ongoing medical conditions, physical restrictions, and cognitive deterioration associated with advancing age.
- Difficulties Maintaining Emotional Health, such as isolation, nervousness, sadness, and loss of a loved one.
Reduced social connections in old age can contribute to feelings of isolation and loneliness, a phenomenon known as social isolation.
Adjusting to Retirement: Retirement can bring about significant lifestyle and identity shifts.
- Existential Concerns: As we become older, many of us wonder about the significance of our lives and the mark we'll make on the world.

The practise of mindfulness can be a useful tool for helping older people cope with these difficulties and flourishing. Some of the reasons why this population should practise mindfulness:

Reducing Stress: 1.

The health, social, and existential stresses that come with ageing can all be mitigated through the practise of mindfulness in older persons.

Controlling one's emotions:

Mindfulness training helps seniors better recognise and manage their emotions, making it easier for them to deal with life's inevitable ups and downs.

Enhanced Coping Capabilities 3.

Fostering a more positive attitude and a willingness to take on new, and maybe, more difficult, ways of coping with life's difficulties.

4 Improved Toughness:

- Through mindfulness, older adults can develop stronger resilience, enabling them to bounce back from setbacks and life upheavals.

Enhanced Social Connection (5):

Mindfulness training can improve interpersonal interactions by increasing compassion, attentiveness, and understanding.

6 Enhanced Mental Performance:

Mindfulness has shown promise in improving cognitive performance and slowing age-related decline, according to certain studies.

Improved Physical Condition ()

Mindfulness has been shown to improve physical health by promoting healthy lifestyle choices including exercise and a nutritious diet.

8. A Stronger Sense of Meaning:

Mindfulness can help seniors find fulfilment by encouraging them to reflect on life's deeper questions.

Mindfulness' Potential Uses in Resolving Aging-Related Problems

There are several ways in which the practise of mindfulness can be used to improve the quality of life for seniors. Some of the many positive effects of practising mindfulness are as follows:

Pain Management: 1.

Reduced pain-related suffering is one way in which older persons can benefit from using mindfulness practises like mindful breathing and body scans for the management of chronic pain.

Emotional Resilience 2. Self-Awareness:

Older adults who engage in mindfulness practises had greater emotional resilience, making it easier for them to deal with loss, isolation, and other issues associated with ageing.

Thirdly, your Cognitive Health:

Mindfulness meditation may benefit cognitive health by increasing focus, memory, and brain plasticity; this is especially true for the elderly.

Tears and Heartbreak (4):

Grieving can be a difficult process, but older folks may find it easier to do so if they practise mindfulness.

Social Isolation (5):

Mindfulness techniques can aid elderly people who are at risk of social isolation because they encourage greater empathy and closer relationships.

6. Spiritual Inquiry:

Spiritual questing is a common activity for the elderly. They can use mindfulness as a means of strengthening their spiritual bonds and expanding their horizons.

Easy Methods to Start Practising Mindfulness Today

The practise of mindfulness can be easily incorporated into the daily lives of seniors. Methods that have proven to be effective include the following:

Mindful Breathing (1):

Maintain a mindful awareness of your breathing. Feel how your lungs expand and contract as you breathe in and out. If you find your thoughts wandering, simply return your attention to your breathing.

Second, a Body Scan:

Scan your body from head to toe, mentally taking stock of how everything is going. Take note of how you feel and pinpoint any areas of stress.

Mindful Meditation (3):

Maintain a daily meditation practise in which you concentrate on your breathing, your body, or a mantra. By quieting the mind, meditating can help one see things more clearly.

4. Exercises in Gratitude:

Affirm your appreciation for the people and events that make your life what it is by setting aside some time every day to do so. A more upbeat disposition may result from this.

Mindful Walking (5):

- Go for a walk in the park or around the neighbourhood and practise mindfulness. Focus on your steps, your environment, and the sensations your body is experiencing while you walk.

Mindful Eating (6):

Think about the food's flavour, texture, and scent as you chew and swallow. Eat at a leisurely pace and undistracted.

Journalists, 7:

- Keep a mindfulness diary to document your thoughts, emotions, and experiences. Keeping a journal can help you recognise your habits and chart your development.

Loving-Kindness Meditation (8):

Sending positive thoughts and feelings to oneself and others is a key component of loving-kindness meditation. This can build self-compassion and empathy.

Mindful Movement: Mindful Movement: Mindful Movement: Mindful Movement:

Practise meditative forms of exercise like yoga and tai chi. Focus on your breathing and how your body feels as you move.

Guided Mindfulness Sessions (10):

- Take part in mindfulness classes taught by seasoned professionals. You may find guided mindfulness activities in a variety of formats, from internet videos to mobile apps.

Beneficial Effects of Mindfulness on Seniors

Positive results can be shown when older persons practise mindfulness:

1. Enhanced Emotional Well-Being:

Practising mindfulness can help with self-control, which in turn lessens the negative effects of stress and sadness.

2. More Stress management: 2.

Mindfulness helps the elderly by providing them with tools for dealing with stress, making it easier for them to deal with daily obstacles.

Better Physical Health (3):

Mindfulness can benefit physical health and reduce the severity of chronic diseases by fostering the adoption of healthful practises.

Increased Social Interaction 4.

Because it encourages compassion and attentive listening, mindfulness is useful for mending broken relationships and combating loneliness.

5. Improved Mental Performance:

Mindfulness may improve older persons' cognitive abilities and memory, according to several studies.

Greater Happiness in Everyday Life:

Increased happiness and a more optimistic view on ageing have both been linked to mindfulness practises.

7. Imperial

A Sense of Meaning:

A deeper sense of fulfilment in later life can be attained via the practise of mindfulness with older persons.

Examples of Actual Achievement

The transformative potential of mindfulness in the lives of older individuals is shown by the following real-world examples:

1. Management of Chronic Pain:

An elderly person with chronic pain uses mindfulness techniques to help manage their symptoms. Over time, people report less pain-related distress and enhanced quality of life.

Grief and Loss 2.

A widowed senior learns to cope with her loss by practising mindfulness. They are able to better understand and cope with their feelings of loss by practising mindfulness.

Social Connection 3.

To practise mindfulness, an elderly person decides to join a support group. Participating in group activities and having meaningful conversations with other members helps members feel less alone.

Conclusion

The benefits of mindfulness on the well-being of the elderly cannot be overstated. Mindfulness helps seniors face the difficulties of ageing with fortitude and a sense of purpose by fostering relaxation, emotional stability, better coping mechanisms, and physical well-being. Mindfulness can have a significant effect on the lives of older persons, both individually and in groups, allowing them to age gracefully and happily. Mindfulness practise in old age can pave the way to a richer, more purposeful senior years.

9.3- Cultural perspectives on mindfulness and mental health

The Effects of Mindfulness on Mental Health: A Cross-Cultural Analysis

Mindfulness, which has its origins in ancient Eastern traditions, is rapidly gaining favour in the West as a technique of improving one's emotional and physical well-being. However, cultural values, beliefs, and practises might affect how the notion of mindfulness is understood and used in the field of mental health. In this article, we'll examine how different cultures see mindfulness and its role in mental health, drawing attention to the many ways in which different societies approach and practise mindfulness and the advantages that may come from doing so.

Culture-Specific Perspectives on Mindfulness

Buddhism has popularised the practise of mindfulness, yet it has its origins in other Asian cultures such as India, China, and Japan. These societies have long adopted mindfulness as part of their spiritual and philosophical traditions. Mindfulness, however, has taken on a variety of forms and interpretations as it has spread over the world.

1. The Buddhist Tradition:

Mindfulness is considered crucial to achieving nirvana in Buddhist teachings. Mindfulness is the practise of paying attention to whatever is happening in the here and now, be it internal or external. Vipassana and Zen meditation, two types of Buddhist mindfulness practise, place a strong emphasis on not being emotionally attached to things.

The Role of the Indian:

In Indian culture, mindfulness is closely associated with the yoga traditions of Hatha Yoga and Raja Yoga. Mindfulness is viewed as a path to enlightenment, self-knowledge, and oneness with the divine.

3. Daoist and Chinese Viewpoints:

Mindfulness in Chinese culture is consistent with Daoist principles like accepting change as inevitable and finding harmony in polarities. Tai Chi and Qigong are two of China's most well-known forms of mindfulness training, and both stress the importance of finding internal balance and connecting with nature.

4. Japanese Zen:

Mindfulness is a central tenet of Japanese Zen Buddhism. Zen practitioners practise mindfulness through activities like tea ceremonies, calligraphy, and gardening.

Modifications for the West (5):

- In Western societies, mindfulness has often been secularised and integrated into therapeutic techniques, such as Mindfulness-Based Stress Reduction (MBSR) and Mindfulness-Based Cognitive Therapy (MBCT). These variants place an emphasis on mindfulness's potential as a stress-buster, emotional-regulation device, and general-health booster.

Mindfulness Practise: Cross-Cultural Differences

The ways in which people of different cultures practise and incorporate mindfulness into their daily lives vary greatly. Some examples of how mindfulness differs between cultures:

One, the debate between collectivism and individualism:

Mindfulness is often embraced in collectivist societies because of its potential to improve interpersonal relationships and group cohesion. However, individualistic societies may place a greater emphasis on the benefits of mindfulness for personal development and insight.

Religious vs. Secular 2.

Mindfulness is welcomed in secular settings for its therapeutic benefits in some cultures, while in others it is practised within a religious or spiritual context.

Formal vs. Informal 3.

Meditation is one way to formally practise mindfulness, but it is also possible to practise mindfulness informally by bringing it into everyday activities like eating, walking, and working. Cultures differ in the ratio of time spent in formal vs. informal settings.

Ritual vs. Silence 4.

- Silence is central to mindfulness practise in some cultures, while ritualistic components like chanting, prayer, and visualisation are more common in others.

Breath-centered vs. body-centered 5.

Body awareness, breath awareness, or both may be included in mindfulness practises. Cultural norms play a role in determining which feature really receives more attention.

The Effects of Mindfulness on Mental Health from a Cross-Cultural Perspective

How mindfulness is understood and practised in the field of mental health is profoundly influenced by cultural norms and assumptions.

The following are some of the most significant cultural views on the connection between mindfulness and psychological health:

1. Eastern Cultures:

Mindfulness is a natural technique to boost mental health and is profoundly incorporated into daily life in many Asian cultures. Meditation, Tai Chi, and yoga are just a few of the favoured methods for calming the mind and body.

Native American Cultures and Practises:

- Indigenous communities worldwide have their own mindfulness practises, frequently anchored in connectedness to the earth, community, and spiritual beliefs. These actions can improve psychological health by increasing feelings of community and belonging.

Integration with the West ()

Mindfulness has become increasingly common in Western therapeutic and clinical settings. It is commonly used as an adjunct to conventional treatments for mental health and has been linked to improved stress tolerance, anxiety control, and general mental health.

African Perspective

Meditation and other forms of mindful movement are commonly used in the spiritual and healing rites of African and African Diaspora communities. It is said that engaging in these activities will help keep the mind and heart in harmony.

Cultural Discrimination 5.

Mindfulness for psychological health is gaining popularity, but its widespread adoption may be contingent on the cultural norms surrounding mental illness and the willingness to seek assistance. Mindfulness can provide a culturally acceptable alternative to obtaining mental health treatment in societies where doing so carries social stigma.

The Pros of Looking at Mindfulness from Different Angles

Embracing cultural ideas on mindfulness can provide various benefits:

1) Cultural Appropriateness:

It's more likely that people will adopt and use mindfulness techniques if they are consistent with their own cultural values and beliefs.

Improved Happiness:

Culturally relevant forms of mindfulness can help people feel more attuned to their communities and more fulfilled in their lives.

Variety in Methods: 3.

Cultures have a lot to offer when it comes to mindfulness practises, so people can pick and choose what works for them.

4. Cultural Competence:

Professionals from culturally and linguistically varied backgrounds are able to give more holistic and compassionate care.

5. International Sharing of Information:

Cross-cultural understanding and knowledge sharing are both enriched when people from different backgrounds share their experiences of mindfulness practises with one another.

Culture-specific examples of how mindfulness is practised in the real world

The wide variety of mindfulness practises in the world is illustrated by the following examples from real life:

1. Kinhin (Japanese):

The practise of walking meditation, or Kinhin, is central to Japanese Zen Buddhism. It embodies the Zen principle of paying attention to the present moment and has strong roots in Japanese culture.

Native American Spiritual Practises That Emphasise Mindfulness:

Mindfulness practises are widely used in Native American healing rituals and ceremonies, where they highlight the need of a strong bond to both nature and community.

Three. Mindfulness-Based Stress Reduction (MBSR):

- Developed by Jon Kabat-Zinn, MBSR is a secular mindfulness programme commonly used in Western societies. It has been modified for use with specific communities and demographics, such as military personnel, healthcare providers, and underrepresented groups.

4. Thai Style Mindful Eating:

Mindful eating is a fundamental part of Thai culture. People who eat thoughtfully focus on the tastes and sensations of the foods they consume.

Conclusion

Our knowledge of and appreciation for this age-old practise and its potential is enriched by cultural perspectives on mindfulness.

advantages for emotional well-being. Since it is both universal and malleable, the practise of mindfulness can easily be adapted to fit into a wide variety of cultural settings. Individuals and mental health professionals alike can benefit from mindfulness's ability to improve well-being, cultivate cultural competence, and advance cross-cultural understanding by adopting cultural perspectives on the practise. Ultimately, mindfulness provides a road to mental wellness that is open to people of all backgrounds and is steeped in the traditions of many civilizations.

Chapter 10:
Beyond the Textbook: Maintaining Your Meditation Practise

10.1- Incorporating mindfulness into long-term mental health maintenance

Integrating Mindfulness into Preventative Care for Mental Health

Taking care of one's mental health is an ongoing process that must be prioritised throughout a person's entire life. Mindfulness has emerged as a valuable tool for long-term maintenance of mental health, however it is just one of many tactics and approaches that can help. It equips people with the tools they need to grow in insight, handle pressure, persevere through adversity, and become stronger overall. In this post, we'll discuss the value of mindfulness training for maintaining mental health over the long term, as well as some concrete methods for doing so and the positive effects they can have.

The Importance of Sustaining Mental Health Over Time

Our mental health is not a fixed quality of our lives but rather a dynamic part of who we are, subject to change as our circumstances do. In the same way that we put time and effort into maintaining our physical health via things like exercise and food, we should do the same for our mental health. Here are some reasons why long-term mental health maintenance is significant:

The

- Preventing mental health problems like anxiety and depression requires regular mental health maintenance.

2. Chronic Disease Management:

Long-term maintenance techniques are crucial for symptom control and general quality of life for people with chronic mental health problems.

3. Constructing Resilience:

The ability to recover from setbacks and obstacles is bolstered by long-term mental health maintenance programmes.

Enhanced Quality of Life:

Taking care of one's mental health is an investment in one's overall happiness and sense of purpose in life.

5. Self-Esteem and Empowerment:

Long-term mental health maintenance encourages people to take charge of their own health and wellness through proactive measures like self-care.

The Role of Mindfulness in Long-Term Mental Health Maintenance

Mindfulness refers to a mental state in which one pays careful, nonjudgmental attention to the here and now. Mindfulness is the practise of paying attention without judgement or reaction to one's internal or external experiences. Mindfulness training is an excellent resource for preserving one's mental health throughout time, as it has been linked to a wide range of positive outcomes. Here's how the practise of mindfulness leads to long-term mental health:

Reducing Stress: 1.

Meditation and other forms of mindfulness practise have been shown to reduce stress and improve mental health.

Controlling one's emotions:

By strengthening one's capacity to recognise and control negative emotions, mindfulness makes it possible to respond calmly and rationally to life's challenging experiences.

Enhanced Coping Capabilities 3.

Reduced reliance on avoidance or other unhealthy coping techniques is one of the main benefits of cultivating mindfulness.

Awareness of Self-Awareness: Awareness of Self-Awareness of Self-Awareness of Self-A

Mindfulness training that is sustained over time has been shown to increase both subjective and objective self-knowledge.

Improved ability to bounce back from adversity

- Mindfulness helps promote resilience, enabling individuals to discover meaning and growth in the face of hardship.

6 Improved Connections:

In order to improve the quality of your interactions, it is important to practise active listening.

7. Enhanced Cognitive Function:

Studies have shown that practising mindfulness can have positive effects on cognition and memory, leading to greater mental acuity and clarity over time.

8. Self-Care Advocacy:
Because it stresses introspection and kindness towards oneself, mindfulness promotes self-care.Methods That Can Be Used Immediately To Improve Your Mental Health

Consistent practise of mindfulness techniques is essential for incorporating it into long-term mental health maintenance. Here are practical strategies for doing so:

1. Daily Mindfulness Meditation:
Set aside some time every day to practise meditation and mindfulness. Start with a few minutes and work up to a few hours. Start with a few seconds and build up to a few minutes.

"Mindful Breathing" (2):
Maintain an attitude of mindful breathing all day long. Spend some time concentrating on your breathing, and refocusing on it if your thoughts wander.

Body Scan 3.
Incorporate regular body scans to check in with physical sensations and areas of tension in the body. Make use of this technique to reduce stress and maintain a strong sense of bodily awareness.

Fourth, "Mindful Walking":

Walking consciously entails focusing on the sensations your feet feel when they make contact with the earth. This is a practise that can be improved by taking a walk in the outdoors.

Mindful Eating (5):

Savour your food by paying attention to how it tastes, feels, and smells while you eat. Don't eat in front of the TV or other distractions.

Journalism (6):
- Keep a mindfulness diary to document your thoughts, emotions, and experiences. Think on what you've learned and how far you've come.

Meditation on Loving-Kindness (7):
You can nurture feelings of compassion and goodwill towards yourself and others by engaging in loving-kindness meditation.

The Eighth Practise of Mindful Movement
Yoga, Tai Chi, and Qigong are just few of the mindful movement practises you can partake in. Focus on your breathing and how your body feels as you move.

8. Unstructured Mindfulness Practise:

- Take part in mindfulness classes taught by seasoned professionals. Mindfulness applications and websites frequently host such classes.

Retreats that focus on practising mindfulness:

Retreats are a great way to immerse yourself in a mindful atmosphere and enhance your practise.

Mindfulness' Long-Term Advantages for Psychological Stability

Long-term benefits of incorporating mindfulness into mental health maintenance include:

1. Constructing Resilience:

Mindfulness training builds resilience over time, making it easier for people to recover from setbacks and see the glass as half full rather than half empty.

2. Improved Emotional Regulation:

The negative effects of stressful emotions on one's mental health can be mitigated with regular mindfulness practise.

3. Enhanced Self-Awareness:

Mindfulness practitioners have a greater capacity for self-acceptance and self-compassion because they get a more thorough comprehension of their own mental processes.

Improved Techniques for Handling Stress:

Mindfulness provides people with long-term, reliable strategies for dealing with stress.

Improved Relationships

Relationships benefit from the improved communication and empathy that comes from regular mindfulness practise.

Enhanced General Happiness (6):

Long-term mindfulness training improves mental health and results in a richer, more satisfying existence.

Long-Term Memory Preservation 7:

Improved memory and mental clarity are only two of the cognitive benefits of mindfulness that can be maintained over time.

Conclusion

Long-term mental health maintenance that includes mindfulness training is a wise choice. Mindfulness training has been shown to improve physical and mental health, as well as overall happiness and well-being. Mindfulness practises, when practised regularly and incorporated into daily life, help people become more resilient, more able to control their emotions, and better able to comprehend oneself. Individuals can better deal with life's difficulties and commit to their mental health in the long run by cultivating a practise of mindfulness.

upkeep of health as a lifelong quest for happiness and satisfaction.

10.2- Resources for ongoing support

A Contents List

1. Set the Scene
2. Instruments for Mental Health
3. Educational Support – Educational Support – a 3rd Educational
4. Tools for Professional Growth and Finding a Job
5 - Financial Help and Backing
6. Help for Families and Relationships
7 Supporting Your Health and Well-Being
8. Community and Social Support
9. Assistance for People with Disabilities and Special Needs
Tenth, Advocacy and Legal Aid
Final Thoughts 11

1. Preface

Having someone there to lean on is fundamental to being human. Life presents us with many obstacles, and in order to overcome them, we often need consistent help from those around us. Mental health challenges, education, professional advancement, money management, relationship maintenance, and health problems all have resources accessible to provide ongoing support and help.

This paper will explore the wide variety of options for continued assistance in several areas of life. We'll talk about all the places people can go to get support, advice, and inspiration.

2. Mental Health Resources

Mental health is a key element of total well-being, and many persons require continuing support to manage their mental health efficiently. Here are some places you can turn for help with your mental health:

a. Therapy and Counselling: Therapists and counsellors can help with many different mental health problems, and they provide services for individuals, couples, and families. Therapists employ a wide range of methods to aid patients in overcoming mental health issues like stress, despair, and anxiety.

c. Support Lines for Mental Health: There are mental health helplines available in many countries that can offer rapid assistance in times of crisis. Helplines like these are usually staffed by knowledgeable people who can provide advice and point you in the right direction for further assistance.

Support groups bring people together who are experiencing similar mental health issues. These gatherings are a great place to make friends, get sound advice, and talk about whatever is on your mind without fear of criticism.

Internet-Based Materials (d) Articles, self-help tools, and guided exercises aimed at improving mental health are just some of the many resources available online and in a variety of apps these days. Some apps even let you have virtual sessions with real therapists.

d. Community Mental Health Centres: All aspects of mental health care, from therapy to medication management to crisis intervention, are available at these facilities. They help people who may not have much money to spare.

EAPs (Employee Assistance Programmes) are a f. As a standard perk, EAPs are provided by numerous companies nowadays. Employee assistance programmes (EAPs) offer private counselling and other services to workers and their loved ones.

3. Aid to Learning

An continual journey to achieve lifelong goals. Some helpful educational materials are included here.

a. Tutoring Services: Tutors and educational centres provide individual and small-group lessons to students of all ages who need extra support in one or more subjects or general academic abilities.

a. Online Learning Platforms: Online platforms like Khan Academy, Coursera, and edX provide a wide selection of courses and tools for self-directed learners.

c. Counselling for College and Career: There are usually counselling offices in both high schools and universities to help students with things like course selection, college applications, and career research.

d. Reference Materials The availability of books, encyclopaedias, and encyclopaedic databases at public libraries can aid students in their studies.

Scholarships and other forms of financial aid, e. Scholarships and other forms of financial aid are widely available from a wide variety of sources to help students pay for college.

b. Adult Education Programmes: Adult education centres offer courses that lead to a high school diploma, a General Equivalency Diploma (GED), or higher education for working adults.

4. Tools for Professional Growth and Finding a Job

Advancing in one's career and getting job might be tough, however there are various services available for continued support in this area:

a. Online Job Boards You can find job ads, networking opportunities, and expert advice on websites like Indeed, LinkedIn, and Glassdoor.

Professional Guidance for Your Future: b. Professional career guidance can be invaluable in helping individuals figure out what they want to do with their lives, what they're good at, and how to get there.

b. Interview Preparation and Resume Editing: Experts in this industry advise job-seekers on how to improve their application materials and ace their interviews.

Workshops for Continuing Professional Education (d) Workshops and courses tailored to individual fields are offered by a plethora of institutions, both offline and online.

d. Professional Development Courses Employment preparation programmes are frequently made available by public and non-profit organisations.

f. Entrepreneurial Resources: The Centre for Entrepreneurial Development offers a variety of courses for persons interested in entrepreneurship and small business management.

5. Help with Money and Other Resources

Maintaining one's financial stability is crucial to one's quality of life, yet some people require constant assistance in this area. Here are some resources available for financial assistance and support:

a. Financial Counselling: Financial counsellors offer advice on money management, debt reduction, and budgeting.

Governmental Helping Programmes (b) The government provides many services to help people who are struggling to make ends meet.

c. Non-Profit Groups Many charitable organisations exist to aid individuals and families in need by providing them with financial aid, grants, and access to financial literacy materials.

d. Credit Counselling: Credit counsellors can assist clients in raising their credit scores and establishing effective repayment strategies for their debt.

a. Investment and Retirement Planning: Financial advisors provide services to help their clients invest their savings properly and prepare for retirement.

f. Financial Tools Available Online: Budgeting, keeping track of costs, and planning for the future are all made easier with the help of a variety of websites and mobile applications.

6. Help for Families and Friends

It is essential for one's health to keep up positive contacts with family and friends. Here are some places to turn for help with domestic issues and friendships:

Family therapists help members of a family figure out how to talk to one another and resolve disagreements peacefully. a.

b. Couples Counselling: Counsellors who specialise in working with couples offer guidance on resolving conflicts and strengthening bonds within relationships.

c. Parenting programmes and Support organisations: Parents experiencing a wide range of issues can find support and direction from programmes and organisations like these.

Services for elderly parents, such as assisted living facilities and carer support, are examples of elder care resources. d. Elder Care Resources.

a. Support for Victims of Domestic Violence and Abuse: Hotlines and other groups offer assistance to people who have been victims of domestic violence or abuse.

Services for resolving conflicts, such as mediation, can be useful for settling disputes within families and between people.

7. Health and Wellness Resources

Taking care of one's body and mind is crucial if one wishes to enjoy life to its fullest. Support your health and wellness efforts with these resources:

a. Primary Care Physicians: Regular check-ups with a primary care physician are critical for preventative healthcare and managing chronic illnesses.

b. Specialist Care: It is crucial to be able to see specialists like cardiologists, dermatologists, and psychiatrists when dealing with complex medical issues.

c. Fitness Centres and Trainers: Gyms, trainers, and exercise classes all work to improve people's health and well-being by encouraging physical activity.

d. Nutritionists and Dietitians: Nutrition professionals can aid people in developing balanced diets and coping with dietary issues.

Apps that promote mental health and wellness e. Mental Wellness Apps: Apps that help with things like meditation, stress management, and mindfulness.

Health insurance helps pay for unexpected medical bills and ensures you can visit the doctor when you need to.

To paraphrase: 8. Community and Social support

Social and neighbourhood

A person's sense of belonging and happiness is greatly aided by the people around them. Some local and online places to turn to for help:

Centres for the Common Good: a. Community centres offer a variety of programmes and activities, from fitness courses to arts and crafts, encouraging social connections.

b. Houses of Worship: Religious organisations offer chances for personal development and civic engagement.

Organisations That Rely On Volunteers (c) Volunteering is a great way to meet new people and give back to your community at the same time.

d. Social Groups (including Meetups): Clubs and websites like Meetup make it easy to connect with people who share your interests.

e. Mentorship Programmes: These programmes pair people with experienced mentors who can help them in many different areas of their lives.

f. Peer Support Networks: Peer support networks bring together people going through similar experiences, such as loss or addiction rehabilitation, to provide each other encouragement and advice.

9. Assistance for People with Disabilities and Special Needs

Individuals with special needs and disabilities typically require continual care and resources tailored to their individual circumstances. In that light, I present the following resources:

A. Offices for People with Disabilities: Students with Disabilities: Many educational institutions and government agencies make accommodations for students with disabilities.

b. Assistive Technology: Assistive hardware and software can provide people with disabilities more freedom to do the things they want to do.

c. Advocacy Organisations: Disability advocacy organisations work to protect the rights and interests of individuals with disabilities.

Disabled people can receive specialised therapies from occupational, speech, and physical therapists. d.

Disabled people and their caretakers can access government programmes that provide them with financial aid and other benefits.

f. Parent and Carer Support Groups: These groups are designed to allow parents and carers of people with special needs a place to meet and talk about their challenges and triumphs, as well as share information and ideas.

10. Advocacy and Legal Counsel

If you or someone you know needs help navigating the legal system or campaigning for your rights, there are services available to provide direction and support.

When individuals or families cannot afford private attorneys, they might turn to legal aid organisations for help. a.

b. Advocacy Groups: Advocacy groups are organisations that aim to improve societal conditions by influencing policy and legislation in areas such as civil rights, immigration, and environmental protection. When it comes to settling disagreements like family conflicts or landlord-tenant disputes, mediation services can be a useful alternative to going to court.
d. Pro Bono Lawyers: Some attorneys provide free legal representation to low-income clients.
e. Government Ombudsman Offices: Ombudsman offices give aid in resolving complaints and issues relating to government agencies and services.

f. Specific Legal Issues Resources: Immigration law, housing law, and employment law are only a few examples of the specialised areas of law for which there are materials available.

11) Concluding Remarks

Persistent encouragement is crucial for success and growth in any endeavour. There is a wealth of information and support networks available to everyone who needs it, whether it's to deal with mental health issues, advance one's education or job, handle one's finances, care for one's relationships, or fight for one's rights.

It's crucial that people know where to find help in times of crisis. To ensure that those who need it can get it, communities, governments, and organisations should keep pouring resources into and increasing access to support services.

Persistent help is proof of the bonds that bind us together as a society. We may all contribute to each other's and society's health and prosperity by giving and accepting help.

10.3- Final thoughts on the mindful journey to better mental health

1. Introduction

In today's fast-paced society, improving one's mental health has risen to the top of the list of priorities. Millions of individuals throughout the world struggle with stress, anxiety, depression, and other forms of mental illness. The stresses of daily life sometimes make it difficult to keep our heads above water. On the other hand, we have access to a valuable resource that can lead us to improved mental health: mindfulness.

Mindfulness is more than a trendy new concept; it's a life-altering discipline. It's a means to better understanding oneself, controlling one's emotions, and thriving in life. This 10,000 word study will investigate the relevance of mindfulness to psychological well-being. We'll take a look at the research supporting mindfulness, its many advantages, and how to start incorporating it into your daily life right away.

Mindfulness in the Digital Age: We discuss the benefits of meditation and its impact on relationships. Additionally, we'll examine how mindfulness can be a beneficial tool in managing certain mental health concerns. A route to greater mental health may be found in this essay, which will act as a full guide to the mindful journey.

2. The Importance of Mindfulness in Maintaining Mental Health

The route to an a better state of health begins with an of the fundamentals. To a of our.

The term "mindfulness" refers to the mental state achieved via paying undivided attention to the here-and-now. To achieve this state, one must be attentive to their inner and outer experiences simultaneously. Accepting our experiences without trying to modify or evaluate them is a central tenet of mindfulness.

Conversely, we can talk about our emotional, psychological, and social well-being when we talk about our mental health. It includes things like our stress tolerance, social skills, efficiency at work, and sound decision-making. The hallmark of robust mental health is not the lack of difficulties, but rather the resilience to triumph over them.

The linked nature of mindfulness and mental wellness is illuminating. Mindfulness training has the potential to be an effective method for improving and sustaining emotional well-being. It equips us with the abilities to handle life's ups and downs, promoting resilience, emotional balance, and a greater awareness of ourselves.

3. Mindfulness and Its Scientific Foundations

Extensive scientific research supports the efficacy of mindfulness in boosting mental health. Mindfulness training has been demonstrated in numerous studies to have beneficial effects on brain structure and function.

The prefrontal cortex, which oversees "executive functions" including decision-making, problem-solving, and emotional regulation, has been linked to mindfulness. Improved cognitive and emotional regulation may result from mindfulness meditation's effect on activation and connection here.

Emotions play a key role in the stress response. Another area of focus is the role of emotions. The amygdala's sensitivity to emotional cues is dampened with mindfulness training, leading to less stress and anxiety.

In addition, the default mode network, a set of brain regions accountable for daydreaming and reflecting on one's own thoughts, benefits from mindfulness practise. Mindfulness training has been linked to reduced activity in this network, which in turn has been shown to lessen the tendency to dwell on the past or worry about the future.

These brain changes coincide with the experiential advantages of mindfulness, including lower stress, enhanced emotional regulation, and increased general well-being.

4. The Upsides of Being Present

The path of mindful improvement to psychological well-being has several advantages. Here are some of the most significant benefits that can be gained through practising mindfulness:

a. Mindfulness is useful for stress management since it facilitates rest and lowers the body's and mind's reaction to a stressful situation.

b. The ability to regulate one's emotions calls for a high level of emotional intelligence, which can be developed through mindfulness practise.

c. Productivity and efficiency gains are possible as a result of mindfulness' ability to improve focus and concentration.

d. The practise of mindfulness leads to increased insight into one's inner world of thoughts, feelings, and actions, which in turn fosters development and acceptance of oneself.

e. The quality of your relationships will improve as a result of your increased capacity for mindful listening and expression.

f. Pain Management: Mindfulness-based practises have been utilised successfully in pain management, helping individuals cope with chronic pain disorders.

g. Mindfulness helps people become more resilient by teaching them how to overcome setbacks and find solutions to problems.

h. The quality of your sleep and the frequency with which you wake up can both benefit from mindfulness practises like meditation and other forms of relaxation.

i. Mindfulness' ability to still the mind and clear away mental clutter has been linked to an increase in both creativity and originality.

j. Increased Quality of existence: Mindfulness has been linked to increased feelings of calm and contentment with one's existence.

These and other advantages make mindfulness an important technique for improving emotional and physical health.

5. Practising Mindfulness on a Daily Basis

The real change happens when mindfulness becomes part of our daily lives, even though its advantages are obvious. Here are some easy methods to start practising mindfulness every day:

a. Take a few moments each day to concentrate on your breathing (also known as "mindful breathing"). Simply observe your breath as it travels in and out, without trying to control it. You can get in some practise whenever and wherever you like.

b. Mindful eating means giving each bite your undivided attention. Give your senses permission to enjoy the meal you're eating. Mindful eating has been shown to improve both meal satisfaction and dietary health.

c. Walking mindfully entails paying attention to each footfall as you go. Take a moment to appreciate your location by sensing the floor beneath your feet, the sensation of motion, and the air around you.

d. Mindful Body Scan: Dedicate some time to scan your body from head to toe, paying attention to any tension or sensations. This method has been shown to reduce anxiety and stress.

e. Mindful Listening: Be an engaged listener in all of your social interactions. Put aside any interruptions and pay close attention to the person speaking.

f. Mindful Journaling: Keep a journal in which you record your feelings, thoughts, and experiences. You can use this to observe your thoughts and feelings and follow your progress towards greater mindfulness.

g. Be aware of how much time you spend on your digital devices. Restriction of screen time and regular digital

cleanse your system and utilise technology more mindfully to reduce stress and interruptions.

h. Mindful Gratitude: Reflect on the good things in your life and actively thank the universe for them every day. Taking up this habit can help you see things in a more optimistic light and improve your outlook on life.

i. Engage fully in mundane activities like washing dishes, brushing your teeth, or taking a shower in order to infuse them with mindfulness.

j. Mini-Mindfulness Breaks: Take frequent breaks during the day to focus on the present moment. Close your eyes, take a few deep breaths, and centre yourself in the present moment.

Mindfulness is an ongoing practise that may be incorporated into any routine. Begin with simple, achievable goals, then add more mindfulness practises as you go. Mindfulness will eventually become an integral part of how you deal with the ups and downs of life.

6. A Walk Through Mindfulness Meditation.

Mindfulness meditation is one of the most effective strategies to develop your concentration and focus. Mindfulness can be cultivated in a systematic way through the practise of meditation, which is a disciplined and intentional activity. In order to help you get started with mindfulness meditation, here is a step-by-step guide:

First, locate a peaceful area.

Find a place where you won't be disturbed and can relax. You are welcome to have a seat on a chair or cushion, or even get comfortable on the floor.

Second, schedule a cutoff time.

Set an objective time limit for your meditative practise. Newbies should aim for 5-10 minutes per session, and they can increase it over time.

Third, establish good posture.

Maintain an upright but relaxed posture, with your hands at your sides. Close your eyes gently, or keep them slightly open with a soft glance, depending on your inclination.

Focusing on the breath is the fourth step.

Focus on the air you're breathing in and out. Feel your chest or stomach rise and fall as your breath enters and exits your nostrils. Breathe as you normally would; there's no need to change anything.

Step Five: Recognise Your Thinking

Thoughts will come up when you meditate. Recognise these thoughts without judgement and return your attention to your breath when they arise. The act of noticing and focusing on one's breathing is fundamental to the practise of mindfulness meditation.

Step Six: Treat Yourself With Compassion

Mind wandering is normal during meditation. When this occurs, you shouldn't be hard on yourself. Instead, be patient and gentle to yourself. You're building awareness muscle every time you return your focus to your breathing.

Step 7: Observe Sensations

Observe the temperature in the room. In addition to the temperature, you can also feel the air movement around you. As a result, you'll feel even more rooted in the here-and-now.

Eighth, finish with awareness.

Take a few deep breaths, slowly open your eyes, and return to your daily routine when you finish meditating. Carry the mindfulness and sensation of presence you cultivated in meditation with you throughout your day.

Consistent use of mindfulness meditation has been linked to significant improvements in psychological and emotional health. Benefits include improved awareness, stress management, and emotional understanding. Your responses to life's difficulties may become more deliberate and balanced with time.

7. Digital Age mindfulness.

Mindfulness has both advantages and disadvantages in today's increasingly digital and interconnected society. Constant notifications, emails, and social media updates can be a source of worry and anxiety, and on the one hand, digital technology can be a source of distraction. However, technology also has the potential to serve as a means of cultivating mindfulness and a boost to our emotional well-being.

The following are some methods for practising mindfulness in the modern world:

a. To avoid mental and physical exhaustion from constant exposure to digital media, try a "digital detox" once in a while. Schedule times during the day when you won't be using any electronic devices.

b. Mindful Tech Use: Instead of aimlessly scrolling through social media or reading emails, practise mindful tech use. Limit purposeful encounters with your digital screen.

c. Apps devoted to helping you cultivate a mindful mindset are increasingly accessible. These applications include guided meditations, clocks, and resources for adopting mindfulness into your regular practise.

d. Join an online mindfulness community or forum to meet people with a similar interest, swap stories, and learn from one another's experiences.

e. Online mindfulness classes and programmes can be helpful because they offer structure and support to their students.

f. Mindful Gaming: Some games and applications are made with the intention of helping players unwind and focus on the present moment. These are some fun ways to bring mindfulness into your free time.

g. If you're going to utilise social media, do so mindfully by following people and communities that encourage reflection, optimism, and development. Maintain a healthy digital lifestyle by carefully curating your space.

h. Use a conscious approach when taking in digital media. Ask yourself if what you're about to click on or read online is in keeping with your own values and health objectives before you do so.

Mindfulness in the digital age calls for a methodical and thoughtful approach to screen time. By employing digital tools wisely, we may harness their potential to enhance our mental health journey rather than impede it.

8. Relationship-Centered Mindfulness

Individual relationships are impacted by our practise, but our practise can also effect our relationships. Mindful communication and presence can improve the way we relate to our friends, family, and colleagues.

Some of the ways in which mindfulness might improve interpersonal connections are as follows:

a. Active Listening: Mindfulness promotes listening attentively to what another person is saying without interrupting them or mentally preparing a response. This creates deeper understanding and empathy.

b. Mindfulness trains you to take other people's perspectives into account when formulating your own response to them. When disagreements happen, you can look at the situation objectively rather than taking a defensive stance.

c. Mindfulness can help you behave more calmly and rationally to stressful events by decreasing your emotional sensitivity to them. As a result, you can reduce tension and foster better relationships.

d. Presence in Quality Time: When spending time with loved ones, practise being totally present. Put down the phone and focus on them without interruptions. Spending time mindfully enhances the value of quality interactions.

e. The practise of mindfulness can help you resolve disagreements in a constructive manner. Arguments can be avoided and peaceful, fruitful conversations can be had instead.

f. Boundaries in relationships are easier to establish and maintain when you practise mindfulness. You learn to better understand and express your own requirements.

g. Practising mindfulness might help you feel more appreciative of the people in your life. Expressing appreciation can deepen friendships and boost the quality of your interactions.

h. Toxic emotions like resentment and fury can poison relationships, but practising mindfulness can make it easier to let them go.

Practising mindfulness in social situations can help you and those around you connect on a deeper, more meaningful level. Careful expression of ideas leads to greater mutual comprehension, sympathy, and friendship.

9. Mindfulness-Based Cognitive Therapy for Disorders of Mental Health

Everyone can benefit from practising mindfulness, but some mental health conditions may find it especially helpful. Let's look at some common mental health conditions and how mindfulness might help:

Anxiety: Practising mindfulness can benefit those who suffer from anxiety by allowing them to worry less and stress out less. Particularly helpful are practises like deep breathing and progressive muscle relaxation.

b. Depression: Mindfulness-based therapies have been demonstrated to alleviate depressive symptoms by boosting introspection and encouraging optimism. The practise of mindfulness can be a powerful tool for overcoming negative thought patterns.

c. Mindfulness is an effective method for dealing with stress. By decreasing the emotional and physical reactions to stress, resilience can be increased by regular mindfulness practise.

d. PTSD (Post-Traumatic Stress Disorder): Mindfulness-based therapies, such as Mindfulness-Based Stress Reduction (MBSR) and Mindfulness-Based Cognitive Therapy (MBCT), have shown promise in the treatment of PTSD by helping individuals process traumatic experiences.

e. Substance Abuse: Including Mindfulness in Addiction Recovery Programmes Can Help People Gain Insight, Control Cravings, and Stay Sober.

f. People with Attention Deficit Hyperactivity Disorder (ADHD) can benefit greatly from mindfulness practises that strengthen concentration and attention. Both executive function and self-control can benefit from these methods.

g. Recovery from an eating problem can be aided by mindfulness-based therapies like Mindful Eating, which encourage a balanced perspective on food and the body.

h. If you suffer from insomnia, you may find that practising mindfulness meditation or other relaxation techniques helps you fall asleep faster and stay asleep longer.

Mindfulness can be a helpful addition to standard treatments for these issues, but it shouldn't be considered as a substitute for professional mental health care. Seek professional help from a mental health expert if you or a loved one are dealing with serious or ongoing mental health issues.

10. Mindfulness: A Way of Life

Improving one's mental health through the practise of mindfulness is not a race to a finish line but rather a way of life. Being mindful is not a goal in and of itself, but rather a mode of being that may and should be developed over time.

Keep these guidelines in mind as you continue your practise of mindfulness:

a. Non-Judgment: Practise non-judgment not only towards external situations but also towards yourself. Being kind to oneself is fundamental to the practise of mindfulness.

b. Realise that developing mindfulness is a process that can't be rushed. Don't give up on yourself just because you've hit a snag or two.

c. Beginner's Mind: As your mindfulness practise develops, maintain the attitude of a newcomer and approach each moment with the same sense of wonder and receptivity.

d. Acceptance: This does not imply that you are giving up your position. Accepting things for what they are and acting accordingly with knowledge and compassion is what this term refers to.

e. The key to mastering mindfulness is regular, consistent practise. Setting up a regular schedule can help you incorporate mindfulness into your life more easily.

f. Integration: Mindfulness is not something that can only be practised during meditation. Try to find ways to apply attention to everything you do.

g. Join a community of people who are also learning to be more mindful. Join a group of people who share your interests and discuss your struggles and discoveries.

h. Mindfulness can lead to personal development and change, so be receptive to the prospect of both. Changes in perspective and outlook on life can be brought about by this experience.

Keep in mind that mindfulness is not a fixed method that cannot be altered to fit your own requirements. The more you practise mindfulness, the more you'll see how it can improve your life in terms of serenity, insight, and happiness.

11. Getting Past Typical Roadblocks

The path towards greater mental health through mindfulness practise is not without its share of difficulties and setbacks. You can use these tests to learn more and improve your practise. Here are some frequent hurdles and techniques for overcoming them:

a. If you struggle to stay quietly or find yourself growing agitated during meditation, it may help to keep in mind that restlessness is a universal human emotion. When unease occurs, bring your attention back to your breathing or your body's feelings.

b. Wandering Mind: This is a common problem for meditators. Don't let this set you back; instead, use it as an opportunity to train yourself to focus on the here and now.

c. Physical Discomfort: During meditation, you may experience physical discomfort, such as stiffness or soreness. Mindfully adjust your posture if necessary, but also see any pain or discomfort as a chance to learn more about yourself.

d. Many people say they can't practise mindfulness because they just don't have enough time. Start with brief, regular sessions; even a few minutes will help. Keep in mind that you can easily include mindfulness into your regular routine.

e. Mindfulness practise may arouse uncomfortable feelings or recollections, which may require you to practise emotional fortitude. Let them bubble to the surface and be seen with compassion rather being pushed down or ignored. Healing and growth are possible outcomes of this procedure.

f. Maintain Mindfulness in the face of adversity is a skill that takes practise. Create a schedule and stick to it, but don't be hard on yourself if you have to skip a session now and then.

g. Let go of preconceived notions of how your mindfulness practise should look and feel. It's not about arriving at some ideal condition, but rather about accepting whatever comes up in the moment.

h. Comparisons: Avoid comparing your mindfulness journey to that of others. It is important to evaluate your own development and happiness as you move forward on your own path.

You can go more confidently and effectively on your path towards mindfulness if you are aware of and prepared to deal with these typical challenges.

12. Learning to Have Kindness for Oneself

One of the most important parts of mindfulness is learning to be kind to oneself. Self-compassion entails showing yourself the same compassion you would show a friend who is going through a tough time.

There are numerous ways in which cultivating self-compassion might improve one's mental health.

When it comes to one's mental health, a holistic approach acknowledges the interconnectedness of each dimension and the importance of nourishing one's overall well-being. Mindfulness acts as a link between these facets of life and encourages a well-rounded and satisfying existence.

15. The Mindful Path: True Stories of Change by Individuals

Throughout our examination of mindfulness and its impact on mental health, it's crucial to recognise the real-life stories of individuals who have gone on this mindful path. Paraphrasing: These transforming accounts give personal attentiveness.

Finding Calm in a World of Worry: Sarah's Narrative

Sarah had a lifelong battle with anxiety. The continual stress and fear of the unknown had taken a toll on her mental health. She tried mindfulness in a last-ditch effort to find some solace. She learned to examine her worried thoughts without judgement through daily meditation and mindful breathing techniques. Paraphrasing began to lessen its grip on my uneasiness. Sarah was able to find serenity within the chaos of her daily life. Mindfulness not only lowered her anxiety but also enhanced her sense of self-awareness and self-compassion.

David's Struggle to Find His Zen

David was a highly successful professional, but he had neglected his health in order to advance his job. He had overextended himself, leading to burnout and tiredness. David, intent on regaining his health, sought out mindfulness practises. He gained the ability to take care of himself and establish limits as a result of his mindfulness training. Every day he meditated and expressed thanks as part of his morning practise. With time, he was able to restore equilibrium in his life. He was able to focus on both his professional goals and his mental and emotional well-being thanks to the practise of mindfulness.

Lena's Story: How Mindfulness Helped Her Recover from a Life-Changing Event

Lena had suffered an emotional trauma that caused her to have recurring nightmares. Traditional therapy had been helpful, but she still couldn't shake the ghosts of her past. She made the choice to learn more about mindfulness as a potential therapeutic technique. Through mindfulness meditation and body scanning, Lena gradually processed her trauma in a safe and non-judgmental setting. As she faced her traumatic past, she practised self-compassion and patience. Lena eventually reached a place of calm and acceptance via practising mindfulness, which allowed her to move on with her life.

These anecdotes showcase the life-altering power of mindfulness in the field of mental health. They show that mindfulness is not a cookie-cutter approach, but rather a flexible method that can aid people wherever they are on their paths to happiness.

16. Conclusion

The path to better mental health through mindfulness is one of introspection, recovery, and development. It encourages us to be fully present in each moment, strengthening our capacity for self-awareness, empathy, and fortitude.

explains the benefits of mindfulness meditation, why it's important in the modern world, and how it affects interpersonal connections.

We also discussed the benefits of mindfulness as a lifelong practise and how it may be used to address particular issues with mental health. We talked about the value of self-compassion and how to overcome common challenges encountered along the path to mindfulness. We also discussed the need of a comprehensive approach to mental health and the part that mindfulness plays in developing resilience.

As we wrap off this investigation, keep in mind that the road to mindfulness is not a straight one. There are times of insight and times of testing. The process calls for persistence, compassion, and a willingness to grow. The path to mindfulness is, in the end, proof that people can change and that they have the ability to enjoy greater emotional and psychological well-being.

To your own mindful journey towards improved mental health, may this investigation prove helpful and illuminating. Keep in mind that there are innumerable others taking their own journeys towards inner calm, fortitude, and satisfaction right alongside you. Hope you keep digging deeper into your inner terrain and expanding your horizons of what's possible in life with the help of mindfulness.

www.ingramcontent.com/pod-product-compliance
Lightning Source LLC
LaVergne TN
LVHW010210070526
838199LV00062B/4525